Quality Assurance and Quality Improvement Handbook for Human Research

Quality Assurance and Quality Improvement Handbook for Human Research

Edited by
Leslie M. Howes, MPH, CIP
Sarah A. White, MPH, CIP
Barbara E. Bierer, MD

JOHNS HOPKINS UNIVERSITY PRESS   BALTIMORE

Johns Hopkins University Press
2715 North Charles Street
Baltimore, Maryland 21218-4363
www.press.jhu.edu

Library of Congress Cataloging-in-Publication Data

Names: Howes, Leslie, editor. | White, Sarah A., MPH, editor. | Bierer, Barbara E.,
    editor.
Title: Quality assurance and quality improvement handbook for human research /
    edited by Leslie M. Howes, MPH, CIP, Sarah A. White, MPH, CIP, and Barbara E.
    Bierer, MD.
Description: Baltimore : Johns Hopkins University Press, 2019. | Includes
    bibliographical references and index.
Identifiers: LCCN 2019001879 | ISBN 9781421432823 (pbk. : alk. paper) | ISBN
    142143282X (pbk. : alk. paper) | ISBN 9781421432830 (electronic) | ISBN
    1421432838 (electronic)
Subjects: | MESH: Clinical Trials as Topic | Human Experimentation—standards |
    Quality Assurance, Health Care—methods | Quality Improvement—standards
Classification: LCC R853.C55 | NLM W 20.55.C5 | DDC 615.5072/4—dc23
LC record available at https://lccn.loc.gov/2019001879

A catalog record for this book is available from the British Library.

*Special discounts are available for bulk purchases of this book. For more information, please
contact Special Sales at 410-516-6936 or specialsales@press.jhu.edu.*

Johns Hopkins University Press uses environmentally friendly book materials,
including recycled text paper that is composed of at least 30 percent post-consumer
waste, whenever possible.

In memory of Cynthia Monahan
and her dedication to the field

Contents

Contributors

Hila Bernstein, MS, MPH
Harvard Catalyst | The Harvard Clinical and Translational
Science Center

Barbara E. Bierer, MD
Brigham and Women's Hospital
Harvard Catalyst | The Harvard Clinical and Translational
Science Center

Elizabeth Bowie, JD, MPH, MSc
Mount Auburn Hospital

Susan Corl, MSW, MPH, CIP, CCRP
Beth Israel Deaconess Center

Jacquelyn-My Do, MPH
Harvard Catalyst | The Harvard Clinical and Translational
Science Center

Lisa Gabel, CIP
Harvard T.H. Chan School of Public Health

Alyssa Gateman, MPH, CCRP
Dana-Farber Cancer Institute

Jennifer A. Graf
Cambridge Health Alliance

Nareg D. Grigorian
Dana-Farber Cancer Institute

Leslie M. Howes, MPH, CIP
Harvard T.H. Chan School of Public Health

Jennifer Hutchinson, CIP, CPIA
Massachusetts Eye and Ear

Cynthia Monahan, MBA, CIP
Partners HealthCare

Eunice Newbert, MPH
Boston Children's Hospital

Sarah A. White, MPH, CIP
Partners HealthCare

Elizabeth Witte, MFA
Harvard Catalyst | The Harvard Clinical and Translational
Science Center

Foreword

As the leader of Public Responsibility in Medicine and Research (PRIM&R), a nonprofit organization dedicated to advancing ethical research, I dedicate much of my time to thinking about how best to support the various components of the human research community in their important work of protecting the rights and welfare of research participants and advancing good science. While there are many resources for institutional review boards (IRBs) and the professional staff that support them, there is very little available to help institutions set up Quality Assurance / Quality Improvement (QA/QI) programs, improve burgeoning QA/QI programs that may already be in place, or codify best practices for QA/QI activities and functions.

In one sense, this is surprising. QA/QI activities touch all aspects of the human research protections program (HRPP). To be sure, the IRB is often thought to be at the core of the HRPP; it is certainly the most visible component. It is no mystery why this would be. Until the 1990s, the IRB was understood to be the primary, if not the sole, entity charged with protecting human research participants. However, after a series of high-profile research scandals came to light in the 1990s and 2000s, resulting in the shutdown of several major research programs, the research community realized that high quality, ethically sound research involving human participants—and the protection of those participants' rights and welfare —must be seen as an institution-wide responsibility, rather than one that starts and ends with the IRB. The idea of the HRPP was born, and, along with it, the need for a mechanism to evaluate and ensure that the HRPP was fulfilling its mission of protecting human research participants in accordance with the federal regulations, local laws, institutional policies, and ethical principles. QA/QI programs emerged to fill this need, as the glue that binds various components of the HRPP together into a functioning, effective whole.

By providing the first comprehensive handbook on QA/QI programs, this book fills a significant gap in the literature supporting the human

research protections field. The timing could not be better. The revised
Federal Policy for the Protection of Human Subjects, or Common Rule,
went into effect on January 21, 2019. This represents the first revision of
the Common Rule since it was promulgated in 1991. One of the most significant outcomes of this regulatory change is the expansion of the types
of activities that no longer require regular IRB review. More specifically,
the revised rule broadens the range of activities that are explicitly defined
as not being research; expands the categories of research exempt from
standard IRB review to encompass more low-risk research; significantly
narrows the range of studies that have to undergo continuing IRB review;
and requires that all domestic, multi-site research centralize regulatory
review in a single IRB of record. As a result of these provisions, it is possible
that a significant portion of research conducted at an institution may not
come before an institution's local IRB for prospective review.

These changes make pressing the need for a strong, well-developed
QA/QI program. With less frequent local IRB review, it will be more important than ever for institutions to have other mechanisms for monitoring
and supporting the quality and integrity of the research activities conducted within their walls. Institutions also need to be confident that investigators and other research stakeholders understand and can operationalize the principles, policies, and regulations that serve to protect the
rights and welfare of human research participants and ensure the integrity
of research. In other words, having a well-functioning human research protection *program*—in which the various components understand their re-
spective roles in promoting ethically sound, compliant, high-quality human
subjects research and work together toward that common goal—is crucial.
A robust QA/QI program, in turn, will serve that goal.

Any institution looking to set up or grow a QA/QI program will want
to consult this volume. It provides clear, concise, practical information
about how to implement, manage, and evaluate a QA/QI program. It is
applicable to all types of institutions: large and small, well-resourced and
resource-limited, and those seeking to set up discrete QA/QI programs as
well as those looking to integrate QA/QI activities within existing offices.
In these pages, readers will find concrete guidance and best practices for
writing and evaluating policies and procedures, conducting investigator
site reviews and IRB evaluations, documenting, reporting, and communicating findings, and creating and providing effective, targeted educational

programs—in other words, resources covering each of the core QA/QI activities.

Just as important as the practical resources included, this book provides invaluable insights and guidance for navigating some of the more challenging aspects of being a QA/QI professional, such as communicating with busy or defensive investigators, maintaining neutrality when reviewing IRB activities that might involve close colleagues, and designing educational programs that are attuned to the needs of various stakeholders. Altogether, the book provides a comprehensive set of tools and strategies for implementing a successful, high-functioning QA/QI program that is tailored to an institution's resources, needs, and culture.

Not only, then, is this the right book at the right time; there is no better group of experts to bring this resource to the QA/QI community. The editors and chapter authors represent national leaders in QA/QI. They have been building, improving, and educating about QA/QI programs for as long those programs have been in existence, and they represent, and lead, some of the most robust and sophisticated QA/QI programs in the country. These experts have been at the forefront of a professional community that has, in the absence of formal programs, been collecting and sharing resources, information, and best practices for many years. In codifying their collective experience and expertise into this volume, Sarah White, Leslie Howes, and Barbara Bierer have provided a great service to the QA/QI professionals who work at the very heart of the human research protection community's collective efforts to advance ethical research.

Elisa A. Hurley, PhD
Executive Director
Public Responsibility in Medicine and Research (PRIM&R)

Preface

Barbara E. Bierer, MD

The purpose of research involving human participants is to develop or contribute to generalizable knowledge; knowledge that will help others to benefit from improved diagnostics, therapeutics, and quality of life. Central to the ability to perform clinical research is the willing participant, an individual who may volunteer for a variety of reasons, including for altruistic reasons. Even when a participant volunteers for access to an investigational product that is not available by any other means, there is no guarantee that the individual will benefit from participation. At its core, clinical research involves a scientific approach to answer a research question, not the provision of medical care.

Clinical research is not, however, without risk, despite investigators' efforts to minimize risk. The majority of research protocols involve some risk, some predictable and some not, and include risks that could impact not only the health and well-being of the participant but their confidentiality, privacy, and dignity. And while potential participants are apprised of reasonably anticipated risks as part of the informed consent process, the risks that are communicated depend upon their predictability and likelihood, and the degree to which the participant understands what is said. And even if risk is fully anticipated and comprehended, adverse events, both anticipated and unanticipated, will happen.

And it is partly because clinical research involves human beings who knowingly put themselves at risk that robust clinical research programs take measures to improve the design, conduct, and oversight of research, and to optimize its protections of human subjects. At a minimum, compliance with federal, state, and other regulations is anticipated, as is compliance with institutional policies and procedures, but, importantly, an institutional human research protection program (HRPP) will develop a system to ensure, not assume, such compliance. That system involves a means to assess ongoing research processes and documentation of both investigator and institutional review board (IRB) activities, including policies, procedures, communications, and files. More importantly, it involves developing a means of learning from its own assessments in order to improve clinical research at the institution more generally, a system that results in continuous improvements in quality, known as quality assurance and quality improvement (QA/QI).

The approach to QA/QI activities in clinical research has borrowed heavily from formal methods developed by QI programs in health and medical care and in other settings. It is instructive to consider how the elements of quality as first defined for health care relate to quality in clinical research. In its treatise, *Crossing the Quality Chasm*, the Institute of Medicine (now the National Academy of Medicine) defined and characterized quality in health care. Quality was defined as "the degree to which health services for individuals and populations increase the likelihood of desired health outcomes and are consistent with current professional knowledge" (232). Six characteristics were described including safety, effectiveness, patient-centeredness, timeliness, equity, and efficiency. Borrowing the application of these terms from health care, all apply to clinical research. Safety, for example, the avoidance of participant injury and harm, is central to clinical research, a focus of and a required element in all protocols, specifically considered by the investigator, and reviewed by the IRB. Equity is embedded in the Belmont Report's principle of justice, ensuring that potential participants have equal access to participation, that there is equitable selection of participants, and that participants of the research should be beneficiaries of the research. Patient- (here participant-) centeredness is at the core of beneficence and the respect for persons.

The approach to QI activities in clinical research involves the systematic review of certain activities, data collection, analysis, and, based on those findings, the introduction of changes—both specific and systemic—to drive improvement in clinical research and the HRPP. There are multiple components to such a system. First, there is the systematic investigation of certain individual events (in health care QI parlance termed "sentinel events") such as problems identified during a review by the IRB. Sometimes investigations into individual events will uncover much larger systemic problems, necessitating changes not only locally but also throughout the institution. Second, periodic, random auditing, data collection and analysis will reveal areas for potential improvement at the site, by the investigator, or for the institution. Any system change will optimally then be subject to further review and improvement. Finally, the overall analysis of the findings across the institution may identify stochastic yet repetitive problems or illuminate areas in need of improvement.

It is important to appreciate that a QA/QI activity need not focus primarily upon whether or not the IRB reviewed and approved a protocol "correctly," nor does it focus upon whether an individual participant fully comprehended the risks and benefits of participation in any given case. The QA/QI activity generally focuses on compliance and on systems and processes. As such, it is a critical tool upon which institutional leadership should depend, producing vital information on the health and vulnerabilities of the HRPP, targets for potential improvement and/or education, and on particular areas (or individuals) of continuing and serious noncompliance. A QA/QI program is, in turn, dependent upon institutional support. Whenever an institution introduces a QA/QI program or activity, human and other resources are needed; critically, the support of institutional leadership is necessary for any suggested changes that result from the QA/QI program.

QA/QI programs initially developed as organic processes driven by the need, occasionally and unpredictably, to audit a person, a program, or a process. Over time, they, like the processes that were the focus of their audits, became more systematic in their approach. They have evolved to become both a core component of HRPPs and an institutional directive, leading to the development of a cadre of QA/QI professionals, trained in auditing techniques, methodology, analysis, communication, and education. Most QA/QI programs in clinical research are local in that they are developed, supported, and operationalized within one institution, one health care setting, or one research unit. But that does not mean that methods, learnings, or tools that are developed need to be or remain local. Indeed, cooperativity among QA/QI professionals has led to progressive improvements in QA/QI activities themselves—a QI approach to QI itself.

This handbook grew out of a sense of shared purpose: QA/QI professionals cooperating to improve the techniques, approaches, and methodologies that they themselves applied. Learning what others had already discovered, adopting those approaches, and then engineering iterative improvements that were again shared with others saved time and resources. It is with this hope in mind—that communicating the shared learnings to date will save time and resources (and frustration and aggravation)—that this handbook was developed. Most importantly, it is our hope that it will lead to improved quality in the protections of human participants, those at the core of research, progress and public health and for whom we are deeply appreciative.

Acknowledgments

This volume would not have been possible without the support of a number of individuals and entities, and we wish to acknowledge them and express our appreciation. First, the listed contributors of the chapters who gathered and organized the content, but also the approach and many of the resources reflect the input of a larger community of QA/QI professionals who have worked together, learned together, and shared experiences and opinions that are, collectively, reflected in this volume. We are grateful to our additional QA/QI subcommittee members, Michele Gomez, Fariba Houman, Grace Kennedy, Angela Lavoie, and Delia Wolf, for their review and support of this handbook. The generosity of our peers, and their commitment to the protection of human participants, is at the core of this handbook.

We also wish to extend our heartfelt thanks to several individuals, without whom this handbook would not have come together. Jacquelyn-My Do made sure that we were all organized, on track and on time; edited our drafts, figures, and tables; collated and formatted the final piece, all with a sense of humor and calm that is enviable. Elizabeth Witte read and reread multiple drafts, edited for clarity, content, and organization, and gave valuable feedback throughout the process. She is the editor extraordinaire. Beyond these two exceptional individuals, Aaron Kirby, Director of Regulatory Affairs and Operations, kept a watchful eye on all of us—and on the calendar—and Evan Sohn, Regulatory Affairs Operations Coordinator, anticipated our every need throughout the process.

The idea for this collection emanated from the QA/QI Subcommittee of the Regulatory Foundations, Ethics, and Law Program of the Harvard Catalyst, part of the Harvard Clinical and Translational Science Center. Harvard Catalyst is generously supported by the National Center for Advancing Translational Sciences, National Institutes of Health Award UL1 TR002541), and financial contributions from Harvard University and its affiliated academic health care centers. The content is solely the responsibility of the authors and does not necessarily represent the official views of Harvard Catalyst, Harvard University and its affiliated academic health care centers, or the National Institutes of Health.

Finally, we are grateful to Johns Hopkins University Press for their help and, importantly, their appreciation of the importance of this contribution.

Note to Readers

This handbook aims to provide human research protection program (HRPP) professionals with a practical guide to create, implement, develop, and modify a quality assurance (QA) / quality improvement (QI) program or function. The handbook is specifically designed for those establishing a new QA/QI program or function and offers several organizational models for consideration. In addition, the handbook provides practical information for improving and strengthening established programs, big and small. The handbook is an evolving document and will be periodically updated as best practices change and emerge.

1

Introduction to Quality Assurance
and Quality Improvement Programs

Hila Bernstein, Jennifer A. Graf,
and Jennifer Hutchinson

History and Evolution of QA/QI Programs

Quality assurance (QA) and quality improvement (QI) programs are a relatively recent development in the context of human research protection programs (HRPPs); their origins can be traced to the late 1990s and early 2000s.

In the late 1990s, institutional review boards (IRBs) and institutions faced increasing scrutiny from the mainstream media, the American public, the US government's Office of the Inspector General, and the General Accounting Office.[1] Criticism centered on instances of failure to obtain prospective IRB approval, minimize risks to participants, obtain legally effective informed consent, provide oversight or continuing review of human research, and minimize conflicts of interest.[2] While some large institutions with well-established, biomedical research programs had already created QA/QI programs,[3] many institutions did not have formal programs or any functional capacity to perform QA/QI activities in place. These criticisms, coupled with discoveries of instances of noncompliance, some of which resulted in serious harm to human research participants, prompted efforts to widely establish QA/QI programs.

In response to the waning public trust in human research, and with the goal of strengthening HRPPs, the US Office for Human Research Protections (OHRP) developed a quality improvement program (QIP).[4] Prior to launching this program, the OHRP evaluated the effectiveness of on-site audits and self-assessments at several institutions. Among the many factors that the OHRP appraised in the development of the program were the confidentiality and sensitivity of information that would be accessed and collected through the QIP. At its core, that information involved primarily personal health information of participants and secondarily information about the investigators and institutions involved in the research. Pilot testing of the OHRP's QIP began in July 2001 and became available to IRBs on a voluntary basis beginning in January 2002; the program was formally launched in April 2002.[5]

The OHRP QIP included three components: QA, QI, and continuous QI. The QA component involved providing an assessment of a program's strengths and weaknesses and evaluating the institution's compliance with federal regulations for human subjects protection. The QI process focused on mechanisms by which a human subjects protection program could improve its operations and better fulfill its intended function. Lastly, the continuous QI portion provided guidance for the continued development of an institution's own QA/QI process.[6] Ultimately, however, OHRP discontinued its QIP program;[7] these functions are now assumed by and embedded within an institution rather than the federal government. However, as a consequence of the QIP model, many, but not all, institutions developed a QA/QI program in order to maintain oversight and quality of its program of human research protections.

The accreditation of HRPPs also fueled the development of QA/QI programs. The largest organization that accredits institutions engaged in human research is the Association for the Accreditation of Human Research Protection Programs (AAHRPP). AAHRPP is an independent, nonprofit accrediting body that uses a "voluntary, peer-driven educational model to ensure that HRPPs meet rigorous standards for quality and protection."[8] Among AAHRPP's current standards for accreditation is the requirement that institutions have procedures in place, which "measure and improve, when necessary, compliance with organizational policies and procedures and applicable laws, regulations, codes and guidance."[9] In addition, institutions should conduct "audits or surveys . . . to assess the quality, efficiency, and effectiveness" of the HRPP to identify strengths and weaknesses and make improvements and monitor quality of a program.[10] Consequently, in order to achieve and maintain AAHRPP accreditation, an institution's HRPP must include elements of QA/QI. Other accrediting bodies have similar expectations.

Today, irrespective of research program size, scope, or accreditation status, many institutions have recognized and embraced the need for, and the utility of, a QA/QI program. Many of these institutions make tools and templates available beyond their own research communities, promoting the sharing of ideas, and in many cases eliminating the need for institutions to duplicate the efforts of others or "reinvent the wheel." Further, a community of professionals engaged in QA/QI activities has developed, and these individuals, often known to each other, serve in both formal and informal consultative roles. As a result, the establishment and maintenance of a QA/QI program or function is feasible even when resources are limited. It is reasonable to expect that, as QA/QI programs become more uniform and robust across institutions, and as researchers incorporate QA/QI activities and suggested best practices into their core research practices, QA/QI functions will exert greater influence on the research enterprise. Ultimately, it is anticipated that this influence will improve the overall quality of research involving human participants and enhance participant protections.

What Is QA/QI?

It is important to differentiate between QA and QI. QA activities involves continuous and systematic monitoring and evaluation of discreet activities to ensure that basic standards are met. The applicable standards will depend on the institution and should include, at minimum, those required by federal, state, and local law (i.e., regulations) and institutional policy. QA activities include assessing investigator compliance with an IRB-approved protocol and program standards. QA may also include evaluating IRB compliance with regulatory requirements and institutional policies and procedures.

To help illustrate QA activities in practice, imagine the National Institutes of Health (NIH) funding a clinical trial involving an investigational drug. At a minimum, such research requires compliance with the Health and Human Services (HHS) Policy for Protection of Human Research Subjects,[11] Food and Drug Administration (FDA) Human Subject Protection Regulations,[12] and applicable NIH policy. Additionally, the regulations set forth by the Health Insurance Portability and Accountability Act (HIPAA)[13] to protect personal health information may be applicable. Applicable state regulations may be more stringent than the federal regulations or address additional expectations, and local ordinances may also apply. Finally, the grantee institution will have its own policies and expectations for human research that must be followed, and those policies are complementary to the federal laws mentioned above. As part of its QA activities, the QA/QI program would audit the ongoing clinical trial to ensure compliance with all of these requirements. The QA/QI program may also provide tools and resources for the investigator and the study team to conduct a self-audit, thereby promoting compliance. While the laws and regulations mentioned above are specific to the United States, all countries have regulations addressing human research, and QA/QI programs are equally important in international settings. Should such research take place outside of the United States, QA efforts would ensure compliance with applicable laws of the host country.[14]

While QA activities may ensure compliance with applicable requirements, QI activities are ongoing efforts that build upon QA activities and are intended to improve the overall efficiency and effectiveness of an HRPP; QI activities may also promote best practice standards and provide tools and resources for both the investigator and the IRB. For example, many institutions elect to apply the International Council for Harmonisation's (ICH) Guideline on Good Clinical Practical (GCP) to human research activities, and the QA/QI program, as a QI activity, may provide model data collection sheets and customizable master logs to assist the investigators in compliance. Further, while the ICH GCP is a routine expectation for the conduct of biomedical clinical trials, it may not be for social-behavioral-education research (SBER) trials. An institution may elect to apply the GCP more broadly to its SBER portfolio. As a result, the institution may expect its SBER investigators to implement a regulatory binder rooted in GCP guidelines. In this specific case, the institution elevates GCP adherence for its SBER community from best practice (QI) to a compliance requirement (QA).

This example helps to illustrate that QA and QI activities run along a spectrum. Applicable laws, regulations, and institutional policies and procedures provide the minimal measures of compliance (QA). From there, an institution may adopt higher standards, as demonstrated above with GCP, for its research portfolio. An institution should be transparent with its community about its compliance measure(s) and provide a rationale when elevating the standard beyond the minimum.

Purpose of QA/QI Programs

QA/QI programs and functions support and advance an institution's efforts to promote investigator and IRB compliance while upholding the overall integrity and quality of human research. QA/QI activities contribute to the central goal of protecting the rights and welfare of human research participants as well as advancing scientifically sound and ethical research. QA and QI activities are core components of any HRPP and are critical to develop and maintain a culture that promotes research integrity and quality. An institution may endeavor to create or revitalize QA/QI efforts to enhance education and outreach, to provide greater support to the research community, and/or to enhance compliance. Particularly in academic and other institutions with large human research programs, QA/QI activities are often executed as an integrated program, often with a distinct component focused on education and oversight within the research community. Some institutions may opt to develop and support a dedicated QA/QI program, implementing key QA/QI functions (e.g., auditing a protocol or investigator) by specific assignment of responsibility to individuals within the organization, commonly within the HRPP office. Often, an institution will develop or reevaluate its QA/QI program or activities in response to a federal inspection or as a corrective action in response to an incident or pattern of noncompliance.

Additionally, as noted above, QA/QI is an important component for an institution seeking to obtain and maintain accreditation by an independent accrediting body (e.g., AAHRPP). An accredited institution must have mechanisms in place to assess compliance with institutional policies and procedures and applicable laws, regulations, and standards; an accredited institution must also have mechanisms to evaluate the overall quality, efficiency, and effectiveness of its HRPP.

Scope of QA/QI Programs

When establishing a QA/QI program, outlining clear parameters for scope of work is essential. It's no surprise that a hallmark of any QA/QI program is its audit function. As a result, initial efforts often focus on the evaluation of investigator compliance. To this end, QA/QI programs develop activities designed to meet these goals, including establishing an audit program and schedule. At a small institution with limited resources, such a program may be modest and include only for-cause audits, whereas a larger, well-resourced, outfit may extend itself further and outline plans for more routine reviews (i.e., not-for-cause audits). As mentioned earlier, those institutions seeking accreditation may look to their QA/QI program to move beyond investigator compliance and evaluate the IRB or larger HRPP. Moreover, although not commonplace today, a program may be able to offer support services to its research community (e.g., external audit preparation, submission assistance, education/training, etc.). The exact scope of an institution's QA/QI program will depend on many things, including the institution's organizational structure, size, resources, and needs. These considerations are discussed in greater detail in chapter 2.

QA/QI Programs in Practice

QA/QI professionals work with other stakeholders in the HRPP and research community, including their IRB counterparts and investigators, to implement improvements based on audit findings, observations, and stakeholder feedback. Therefore, QA/QI professionals should endeavor to build strong, collaborative relationships with relevant departments and investigators, while preserving their objectivity and independence. This is often a difficult balance to achieve, as the QA/QI professional is not only a colleague but is also evaluating and judging investigators and IRB administrators.

The knowledge base of a QA/QI professional is extensive. QA/QI professionals must be familiar with current institutional policies, most notably those of the IRB, as well as research administration, the clinical trials office, privacy and information security office, investigational drug service, and others. Serving as a catalyst for institutional and investigator compliance, QA/QI professionals may provide comments or recommendations regarding potential policy modifications based on their findings and/or the needs of the research community, or when policies are internally incompatible.

A QA/QI program's success depends upon the support of institutional leadership and the research community as a whole. Institutional commitment to quality and excellence in this area is particularly critical. For this reason, fostering collaborative relationships with institutional stakeholders is key to the development, implementation, and maintenance of any QA/QI program.

SUMMARY

- QA involves continuous and systematic monitoring and evaluation of discreet activities to ensure that standards are met and that the organization's policies and procedures as well as national, state, and local laws and regulations are followed.

- QI activities are intended to build upon QA activities to improve the overall efficiency and effectiveness of an HRPP and may also promote best practice standards.

- QA/QI programs support and advance an institution's efforts to promote investigator and IRB compliance, while upholding the overall integrity and quality of human research.

- QA/QI professionals should work with other stakeholders in the HRPP and research community to implement improvements based on audit findings, observations, and stakeholder feedback.

- Institutional support of the QA/QI program and its commitment to quality and excellence are particularly important for success.

REFERENCES

1. Office for Human Research Protections, "Objectives and Overview of the OHRP Quality Improvement Program."

2. Office for Human Research Protections, "Objectives and Overview of the OHRP Quality Improvement Program."

3. University of Pittsburgh, Education & Compliance Office for Human Subject Research, established in 1996.

4. Office for Human Research Protections, "Objectives and Overview of OHRP Quality Improvement Program."

5. Office for Human Research Protections, "Objectives and Overview of OHRP Quality Improvement Program."

6. Office for Human Research Protections, "Objectives and Overview of OHRP Quality Improvement Program."

7. Office for Human Research Protections, "OHRP QA Self-Assessment Tool."

8. Association for the Accreditation of Human Research Protection Programs, Inc., "Our Mission."

9. Association for the Accreditation of Human Research Protection Programs, Inc., "AAHRPP Evaluation Instrument," 52–55.

10. Association for the Accreditation of Human Research Protection Programs, Inc., "AAHRPP Evaluation Instrument," 52–55.

11. US Department of Health and Human Services, "Policy for Protection of Human Research Subjects."

12. US Food and Drug Administration, "Regulations: Good Clinical Practice and Clinical Trials."

13. US Department of Health and Human Services, "Summary of HIPAA Privacy Rule."

14. Office for Human Research Protections, "International Program."

2

Types of QA/QI Programs:

A Review of Three Models

Jennifer A. Graf and Jennifer Hutchinson

Purpose

This chapter focuses on three common models for executing QA/QI responsibilities:

1. Independent QA/QI program
2. QA/QI function within an IRB office or unit
3. External QA/QI expert

While creative alternatives may be necessary or desirable to establish a QA/QI program or function, these three approaches are the most prevalent organizational models for QA/QI. When evaluating which model to implement, key issues to consider are the size of the institution's research program, the type of research conducted at the institution, the needs of the research community, available human and financial resources to establish and maintain the program, and importance of maintaining objectivity and neutrality.

QA/QI Model Parameters

The prevailing characteristics, suggested reporting structure, advantages, and disadvantages associated with each model are outlined below. Some of these characteristics are not unique to a particular model, but they are important to consider when determining the appropriate model for an institution. A summary of the models can be found in Table 2.1.

When introducing any QA/QI model, an organization should be cognizant of any established and dedicated compliance unit(s) that may intersect with human research. Oftentimes, these units have a specific area of focus,

Table 2.1. Common models of QA/QI programs

Model	Characteristic	Reporting Structure	Advantages	Disadvantages
Independent QA/QI program	Separate, distinct from IRB and other HRPP-related offices *Note: QA/QI director and IRB director commonly report to the same individual*	QA/QI staff typically report to HRPP director or IO *Note: QA/QI director and IRB director commonly report to the same individual*	• Permits objective, 360° evaluation of entire HRPP, including the IRB • Minimizes overlap or preoccupation with functions of other HRPP offices • Allows QA/QI staff to provide education and support services • QA/QI staff can focus on professional development, education, and training specific to QA/QI activities	• Clear definition and communication of scope are essential to prevent overlap with other offices • Financial position of institution must be sufficient to provide and maintain staff, space, and support • Requires ongoing communications with HRPP offices to ensure QA/QI personnel are kept abreast of policies
QA/QI function within IRB unit	Individual(s) within IRB (e.g., IRB administrator or staff member) provide dual QA/QI and IRB services	Individual(s) typically report to IRB director/administrator *Note: Reporting hierarchy typically remains within IRB operations unit*	• Requires little or no additional cost or staff • Personnel designated to perform QA/QI activities may have requisite regulatory knowledge and be knowledgeable about institutional IRB policy and process	• Existing IRB personnel may not be qualified and/or sufficiently experienced to perform QA/QI activities; may lack experience conducting research • Day-to-day workload of IRB staff may not permit time for QA/QI • Investigator apprehension / fear of bias if IRB staff performs both IRB and QA/QI duties • Potential COI due to dual roles • May create workplace tension when performing QA/QI IRB reviews (e.g., reviewing IRB colleague's or supervisor's work)
External QA/QI expert or program	Individual(s) or organization(s) hired on contract basis to perform specific task, provide opinion on project/situation, etc. *Note: Hired for professional expertise and specialty in the field*	Varies depending on the scope of work specified in consulting agreement *Note: May report to IO, a designated HRPP official, General Counsel, or oversight/steering committee*	• Allows for a 360° evaluation of HRPP • Consultant is likely experienced in conducting audits and providing feedback to institutions • Consultant is seen as unbiased and a neutral party	• Consultant fees and structures vary; may be costly • Not a long-term solution for offering QA/QI support and education services • Consultant(s) lack familiarity with institutional policies, procedures, and practices • Absence of established relationships with investigators and staff • Confidentiality of PHI

e.g., cancer-related research, pharmacy, research misconduct, laboratory and biosafety. Before unveiling a QA/QI program, an organization should first identify each existing and applicable compliance unit and take note of its scope and authority in relation to the QA/QI program. This will ensure QA/QI activities are well directed and do not duplicate existing efforts. Establishing a relationship with existing compliance units from the onset will help to foster collaboration across units; this may include conducting joint audits, developing a cross-unit escalation plan, and sharing best practices, e.g., tips for engaging the research community.

Independent QA/QI Program
Characteristics

In the independent QA/QI program model, the QA/QI program is independent from IRB operations and all other HRPP-related offices (Figure 2.1). Excellent communication and clear definition of scope are essential to prevent overlap with other offices and to facilitate coordination, as appropriate.

Reporting Structure

The program may be established within the same office as the IRB operations unit (e.g., Regulatory Affairs, Research Administration, Human Research Protections Office), but the QA/QI program must maintain staff independent of the IRB staff and must have a separate reporting hierarchy. QA/QI staff typically report to the HRPP director or institutional official (IO). It is common for the QA/QI director/administrator and the IRB director/administrator to report to the same individual.

Advantages
- The independence allows for an objective and comprehensive evaluation (sometimes referred to as a "360° review") of the entire HRPP, including the IRB.
- The program's primary focus is on QA/QI activities, minimizing the potential for preoccupation with, or duplication of functions with, other HRPP office and IRB operations.
- The independent QA/QI program may offer a broader range of services than other models, including a focus on education and support services.

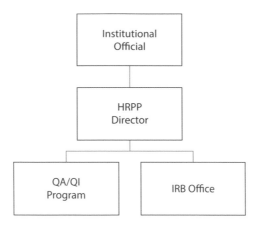

Figure 2.1. Independent QA/QI Program

- Given that the QA/QI staff are not involved in IRB review or approval of protocols, an independent QA/QI program may foster a sense of collaboration with investigators by providing research assistance and support. This may help dispel a frequent misconception among researchers that QA/QI programs are strictly compliance enforcement entities, and may, in turn, encourage investigators to work collaboratively with QA/QI staff.

Disadvantages
- Establishing an independent QA/QI program/unit requires significant resources. To implement and sustain this model successfully, the institution must have the financial resources to provide and maintain adequate staff, sufficient space and infrastructure, and ongoing support to meet institutional needs.
- Independent programs must maintain careful and ongoing communications with the IRB office, clinical trials office, etc., to ensure that personnel are kept abreast of policies and preferred practices and to coordinate efforts as appropriate.
- For voluntary program functions, additional effort may be necessary to engage investigators and to implement proposed corrective actions and/or best practice recommendations.
- Hiring and retaining competent and experienced staff may be a

challenge, as qualified professionals in this field can be difficult to recruit, identify, and retain.

The independent QA/QI program/unit is often considered to be "the gold standard," given its independence from other offices; however, the human and financial resources required to establish and maintain such a program may be prohibitive for some institutions. Furthermore, the size and/or scope of an institution's research portfolio may not necessitate such a robust framework.

QA/QI Function within IRB Unit

Characteristics

In the model in which the QA/QI function is embedded within an IRB unit or office, the QA/QI program is typically smaller (e.g., 1–2 staff members); this model is particularly relevant for institutions with smaller research portfolios or restricted research activities (Figure 2.2). An individual(s) often provides both QA/QI and IRB services (e.g., an administrator who is responsible for both QA/QI activities and certain IRB operations, or an IRB staff member who may do some QA/QI activities for a percentage of their time).

Reporting Structure

The reporting hierarchy in this model typically remains within the IRB operations unit, with QA/QI staff reporting directly to the IRB director/administrator.

Advantages
- May require little or no additional cost or staff.
- Personnel designated to perform QA/QI activities typically already have the requisite regulatory knowledge and are also knowledgeable about institutional and IRB policies and processes, etc.
- Investigators and their research teams are often familiar with and known to the QA/QI-IRB staff. Quality improvement activities can often be introduced early in the conduct of a trial, since all investigators will engage with the IRB prior to initiating any human subjects research.

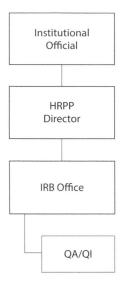

Figure 2.2. QA/QI function within IRB Office

Disadvantages

- Given the relationship of the IRB to QA/QI functions (and the fact that often the same person is functioning in both capacities), it is exceedingly difficult for the person charged with QA/QI responsibilities to audit, monitor, or evaluate the IRB itself. This limitation is important to recognize from the outset, and other provisions for evaluating, maintaining, and improving IRB quality and operations should be considered.
- Existing IRB operations personnel may not be qualified and/or sufficiently experienced to perform QA/QI audits. If those who perform QA/QI activities lack prior experience, it may limit their effectiveness and negatively impact the validity and utility of the findings.
- Given the overlapping responsibilities, and due to potential conflict of interest (COI) and/or bias, the individuals charged with conducting QA/QI activities may have difficulty maintaining objectivity (see discussion on Neutrality and Objectivity below). This is particularly true for activities involving oversight of the IRB office.
- Given the dual nature of the QA/QI and IRB role, an investigator may be reluctant to be forthright with staff performing QA/QI activities

due to fear of bias when the staff performs IRB-related work involving the investigator's research or exposure of noncompliance. It is also possible that the opposite type of relationship may develop. A staff person with dual QA/QI and IRB responsibilities could be perceived as being too close to an investigator and giving preferential treatment to the researcher and/or research team.

- Depending on the size of the program, the day-to-day workload of an IRB operations unit may not afford a staff person the time required for meaningful QA/QI work. As a result, QA/QI activities may be perceived as reactive, addressing noncompliance, rather than proactive, devoted to training, education, and the development of tools and resources.

The model of a QA/QI program embedded within an IRB office is common among smaller institutions and/or when resources are limited. While challenges exist, including managing potential COI and/or bias, a QA/QI function operating under this model may be effective and may offer significant efficiencies.

External QA/QI Expert

Characteristics

In the external QA/QI Expert model, an individual(s) or organization(s) is employed independent of the institution and is hired on a contract basis (Figure 2.3). The consultant(s) may perform a specific task, provide an opinion as to how to proceed with a particular project or situation, or recommend a proposal or plan to address a particular situation. The person or organization is selected and hired based on expertise and qualifications in the field, and the selection may change depending upon the context and need. Occasionally, a smaller institution will contract with a large, often nearby, entity with a QA/QI program for intermittent services. Such an arrangement avoids the need to find an external consultant and provides for developing a single contract, one that addresses issues such as reporting responsibilities, confidentiality, records retention, etc.

Reporting Structure

Reporting structures vary depending on the scope of work specified in the consulting agreement or institutional agreement with the IRB. The

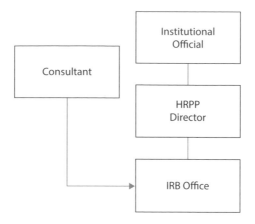

Figure 2.3. External QA/QI Expert or Program

external QA/QI expert may report to the IO, a designated HRPP official, general counsel, or an oversight/steering committee.

Advantages

- Engaging an external QA/QI expert independent of the institution allows for an objective, comprehensive, external evaluation of the entire HRPP or any component thereof.
- An external QA/QI expert is likely to be experienced in navigating complex and challenging conditions (e.g., introducing a new QA/QI service, conducting a for-cause external audit, or preparing the institution for an FDA inspection). The external consultant is focused on QA and QI and will have expertise in conducting audits and providing feedback to the institution. In the case of investigator audits, the institution is then in a position to decide whether the institutional representative or the consultant will provide feedback to the researcher.
- Investigators, HRPP staff, institutional officials, and others typically perceive an external QA/QI expert as an unbiased and neutral party.

Disadvantages

- Fees for a QA/QI expert vary but tend to be costly, especially if hired at a consultant rate.

- QA/QI expert consultants are frequently engaged for specific, time-defined projects and, therefore, do not provide an institution with a long-term solution for offering QA/QI services and support to the research community.
- QA/QI expert consultants often lack institutional context, including familiarity with institutional culture, policies, procedures, and practices.
- QA/QI expert consultants often do not have established, long-term relationships with investigators and staff. (This may also be perceived as a potential advantage.)
- If an institution is subject to HIPAA, then a business associate agreement must be executed to maintain the confidentiality of protected health information.

Given the potential costs associated with the external QA/QI expert consultant model, hiring an external QA/QI expert may not be a viable or sustainable option for many institutions. That said, the consultant does provide a uniquely independent perspective and may best be deployed on a case-by-case basis when particular expertise is required and not available within an institution. It should be noted that an external QA/QI expert consultant may complement rather than replace an institutional QA/QI program in specific situations, when additional review, support, or expertise is desired.

Neutrality and Objectivity

When considering a QA/QI model to adopt, it is important to consider the neutrality and objectivity of a QA/QI professional and to evaluate whether and how competing interests or bias may influence judgment and decision-making.[1] Asking QA/QI professionals to fulfill dual roles may create awkward or uncomfortable situations and/or conflicting interests that may negatively impact the integrity of the review and monitoring process and possibly the QA/QI program as a whole.

For example, a QA/QI professional who reports to the IRB director may be reluctant to identify deficiencies or make suggestions for improvements within IRB operations. This dynamic could also introduce tensions if, for example, the QA/QI professional finds and must report deficiencies related to the work of a colleague that may impact the colleague's standing or professional advancement. A more problematic situation arises when the deficiency is related to the work of or oversight by the IRB director. A QA/QI professional who is also an IRB reviewer may face similar challenges. If the individual helps a study team prepare an IRB submission and then is assigned to review the submission and/or participate in IRB deliberations, legitimate and serious questions may be raised about the objectivity and independence of the review. Consideration of how to segregate potentially necessary and helpful investigator assistance from the IRB review itself is, therefore, important.

When a conflict is present, it is important to consider ways to minimize, mitigate, or eliminate the conflict and/or bias. Consider, for example, a QA/QI professional who is involved in the prereview or review of an IRB submission and is then later asked to perform an audit of the same study; the individual should disclose this potential conflict before the audit and in the report of findings. However, merely disclosing a potential conflict does not mitigate or eliminate the conflict; if possible, the prudent course of action would be to eliminate the potential conflict by having another qualified staff person conduct the review.[2] Care should be taken to avoid any perception that either the program or an individual staff member may favor a particular individual or group (i.e., an investigator, study team, IRB). Use of standardized, objective tools (e.g., audit tools, template reports) may also aid in maintaining objectivity and are described further below.

Considerations in Hiring a QA/QI Professional

The identification and recruitment of QA/QI professionals, especially those with previous direct QA/QI experience, is challenging. Instead, institutions may favor incumbents with various backgrounds and expertise. For example, recruiting an experienced IRB administrator for a QA/QI role would ensure that the QA/QI professional possesses the requisite knowledge of applicable regulations and IRB operations. A clinical research study coordinator or project manager would have demonstrated their ability to support an investigator or research team successfully, which is an asset in serving a research community. Alternatively, past experience in industry, including with a pharmaceutical company, device company, or contract research organization, could provide experience related to FDA-regulated studies and an understanding of study management from a sponsor perspective. In addition, a candidate who has previously conducted human research would be knowledgeable about the intricate operations of carrying out a research study, which is advantageous for an auditor.

Independent of an incumbent's prior experience, a QA/QI professional should have or be required to develop extensive knowledge and understanding of applicable laws, regulations, and policies governing human research. Ideally, a candidate possesses these prerequisites upon hire. If not, however, a new staff member should learn these skills and competencies on the job while developing an appreciation for institutional policies, procedures, electronic systems, and institutional culture. Perhaps equally essential is the ability of a QA/QI professional to solve problems, make decisions, provide clear communication, and adapt to change. These interpersonal skills are key ingredients that allow an individual to thrive while auditing, delivering difficult findings/observations, liaising between the IRB and investigator, and/or providing respectful and responsive customer service. A sample job description is given in Appendix B.

SUMMARY

- Three common QA/QI models are (1) an independent QA/QI program; (2) a QA/QI function within the IRB office; and (3) an external QA/QI expert.

- An independent QA/QI program operates independently from the IRB and other HRPP-related offices.

- A QA/QI function within the IRB office has IRB staff members who provide both QA/QI and IRB services.

- An external QA/QI expert is independent of the institution and is hired on a contract basis.

- Each QA/QI model has its advantages and disadvantages; every institution must determine which model best suits its needs, based in part on scope, size, and complexity of the human research program.

- Consideration of the neutrality and objectivity of QA/QI professionals is important when evaluating which QA/QI model is best suited to the institution's needs.

- A QA/QI professional should have a solid understanding of applicable laws, regulations, and institutional policies governing human research.

REFERENCES

1. E. Emanuel, *The Concept of Conflicts of Interest*, 758–66.
2. E. Emanuel, *The Concept of Conflicts of Interest*, 758–66.

3

Policies and Procedures

Barbara E. Bierer and Eunice Newbert

Purpose

Like all institutional programs, leadership will establish the roles, responsibilities, and authorities of an institutional QA/QI program. The QA/QI program itself should develop and then comply with policies and procedures that outline how the QA/QI individuals will execute those assigned roles and responsibilities. In addition to the policies and procedures of the QA/QI program, it is equally important for QA/QI program personnel to identify and understand the policies and procedures for other programs and departments within an HRPP, which, taken together, provide the overall framework for ensuring human research subject protections.

This chapter defines and distinguishes between policies and procedures and discusses their development, design, and utility within a QA/QI program. This chapter also addresses the relationship between policies and procedures implemented by institutional leadership, and the laws, regulations, and guidance enacted and enforced by regulatory agencies.

Overview

A major responsibility of any QA/QI program is to help ensure that institutional policies and procedures are consistent with national and local laws and regulations, and that employees and staff understand and follow these laws, regulations, and policies. A principal responsibility of QA/QI personnel is to audit—and educate—with these directives in mind, so understanding the differences between them is essential. The general differences between laws, regulations, guidance, policies and procedures are given in Figure 3.1.

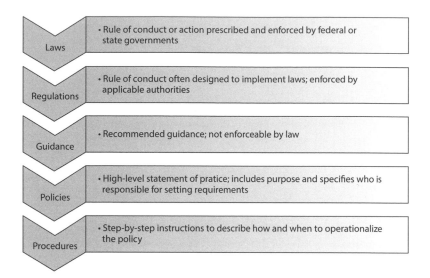

Figure 3.1. Characteristics of Laws, Regulations, Guidance, Policies, and Procedures

Laws, Regulations, and Guidance Documents

A law is a rule of conduct or action prescribed and enforced by the federal or state governments. A regulation is a rule or order that carries the same force as law but is issued and enforced by an executive authority or regulatory agency of the government. Regulatory agencies adopt regulations to monitor and enforce laws.

Guidance documents are not enforceable by law. Instead, they are statements from regulatory agencies that represent the agency's current thinking on a topic related to either existing laws and regulations or questions that have arisen. In general, alternative approaches to the guidance may be taken, but individuals or institutions are encouraged to contact agency staff to discuss such approaches before implementing them. In addition, documentation of the alternative approach, agency communications, and the reasons for preferring the alternative are suggested. Institutions should consider guidance documents when developing policies to assist in the interpretation of applicable laws and regulations. See Table 3.1 for examples of federal documents.

Table 3.1. Examples of federal documents related to IRBs

Document Type	Example
Law	Congress National Research Act (1974)
Regulation	Protection of Human Subjects: 21 CFR 50 (FDA) 32 CFR 219 (Department of Defense) 38 CFR 16 (Veterans Health Administration) 45 CFR 46 (HHS)
Guidance	OHRP/FDA: Institutional Review Board (IRB) Written Procedures: Guidance for Institutions and IRBs (May 2018)

The Purpose of Policies and Procedures

While laws and regulations are rules used to *compel* or enforce behavior, policies are principles used to *impel* or guide behaviors toward a specific goal or outcome. Policies are a course of action applicable to the institution or organization. While they do not directly carry the same force of laws, policies must conform to and comply with existing federal, state, and local laws and regulations. An institutional policy may, however, go "beyond" the law and impose additional responsibilities, limitations, or actions. For instance, neither the law nor regulation requires the IRB to review quality improvement activities. The institution may, however, designate the IRB as responsible for determining whether an activity is QI or research, thereby imposing a requirement upon its employees (investigators, clinicians, staff) to present any planned activity to the IRB for a determination. Any violation of institutional policy by an individual may result in consequences, such as retraining, warning, or personnel changes. However, any violation of law or regulation by an individual may result in federal or state penalties, including fines. Policies and procedures help staff comply with the expectations of the institution and the professional expectations of their jobs. The differences between policies and procedures are summarized in Table 3.2.

Policies

Policies are high-level statements that set the strategic tone for an institution or organization. They are used to guide decisions by stating, with clarity and transparency, both *what* course of action should be followed

Table 3.2. Distinguishing between policies and procedures

	Policy	Procedures
Defined as	A course or principle of action adopted or proposed by a government, party, business, or individual	Detailed, step-by-step instructions to operationalize a policy
Statements of	*What* an institution does and *why*, including purpose and background	*How* and *when* to operationalize a policy
	Who is responsible for setting policy	*Who* is responsible for operationalizing
Expressed in	General and broad terms	Specific details

and *why*. Policies often specify *who* (the individual or group) is responsible for executing the policy. Procedures, on the other hand, are detailed instructions of *how* the responsible parties should operationalize the policy.

A policy is a high-level statement of practice that has been developed to reflect the institution's mission and objectives and is communicated as an expectation of institutional leadership. Policies are developed to establish what course of action to follow and to provide the background and framework to help institutions make difficult decisions and enforce rules.

The included elements may differ depending upon the purpose of the policy but will generally include the following:

- Policy statement: *what* the policy is and a description of its intended purpose
- Purpose: *why* the policy is required
- Applicability and scope: to whom and to what the policy applies
- Substance of the policy: limitations and expectations
- Applicable laws and regulations to which the policy is responsive, if applicable
- Responsibilities: *who* is responsible for policy execution and enforcement
- Who approved the policy
- Date of approval

Policies provide a means to protect the legal interests of an institution and its employees and define the rights and obligations of both the institution and its employees. Policies should strive to be clear and transparent, to treat all involved parties fairly, and to conform to local, state, and federal laws and regulations.

Generic Policy Outline

- Title
- Outline of the policy
- Source of review and approval ("Approved by")
- Date of approval
- To whom the policy applies
- Policy:
  - Introduction
  - Scope and organization of the policy
    — What the policy governs
  - Why the policy is needed
  - Terms used
  - Responsibilities and obligations of the various affected parties
  - Rights of the various affected parties
  - Policy-specific sections
  - Practical implementation considerations (see "Procedures")
  - Compliance expectations
  - Consequences of noncompliance, if applicable
  - Dispute resolution, if applicable
  - Applicable laws and regulations

Procedures

While policies lay out what management wants employees to do, the procedures describe how the responsible parties should operationalize the policy. Procedures are step-by-step instructions that optimize the likelihood that the policy will be carried out in a standard fashion and help each individual within the organization act consistently and predictably.

Procedures should be envisioned as a living document: whenever an unanticipated question or new issue arises, the procedure should be reviewed, annotated, and revised as appropriate. While procedures can be embedded in policy documents, they are more usually presented as separate documents. Procedures rarely require the level of review and approval by the institution that are required of policies. Since that process can be lengthy and burdensome (and can sometimes serve as a disincentive to make helpful changes), procedures that track to, but are separate from, institutional policies are recommended. Procedures can take a variety of forms. Sometimes the instructions include a detailed list of expectations that track from the beginning to end of the process. Forms or checklists can be useful to ensure that all steps are completed and to document that a procedure has been carried out according to policy. For example, the procedures for an audit policy may include the use of a review/audit/monitoring checklist. If a form or checklist is required for documentation, these forms should be referenced within the procedure (not the reference policy) document itself, either with a citation (e.g., web link) as to where to find the form or checklist or included therein.

Policies and Procedures for QA/QI Programs

As stated previously, the fundamental role of a QA/QI program is to assure institutional leadership, through monitoring and reporting, that programs and departments comprising the HRPP have developed, implemented, and are complying with institutional policies and procedures, and applicable federal and state laws and regulations.

Individuals responsible for execution of the QA/QI program will be guided in their work by an institutional policy that outlines the QA/QI program itself, as defined by leadership. That policy should outline the roles and responsibilities of the QA/QI program, including its scope of authority and limitations thereof and reporting structure. Procedures may give further specificity. QA/QI management and staff should understand and agree with the scope and responsibilities as outlined; all questions and ambiguities should be clarified with leadership and documented.

Recommendations for what might be included in a model QA/QI policy manual are given in Appendix B.

Written thoughtfully, policies and procedures can facilitate consistency, build trust, foster transparency, and serve as an effective method of documenting processes. Policies and procedures document a QA/QI program's practices in writing so that they are available for reference. Further, they serve as a valuable teaching tool for new staff members, leadership, and researchers. A manual of procedures, including descriptions of all necessary steps, reduces variation, complexity, and speculation and guides QA/QI staff members in their actions and during audit proceedings. Procedures such as selecting sites to visit, notifying investigators of difficult news, and making determinations regarding reporting events, and reporting responsibilities and timing, help reduce any sense that an individual or program is "targeted" or that the QA/QI staff is capricious in its actions. Procedures help to legitimize and support QA/QI staff who are often placed in difficult positions with respect to investigators and their study teams, with whom they need to interact in the moment, for a specific audit or action, and in the future. Explicit policies help to standardize and professionalize—and depersonalize—QA/QI determinations, especially those that result in unfavorable actions.

Policies and procedures facilitate consistency among staff responsibilities, expectations, and actions in a research team, a division, or a department. The clarifications provided within policies and procedures can help faculty and staff understand their roles and responsibilities as well as those of others, within predefined limits. Well-written and well-conceived policies and procedures help to establish clear expectations, define programmatic boundaries, and routinize operations while increasing efficiency. Interestingly, effective policies and procedures may also help to reduce anxiety and apprehension associated with unanticipated audits, correspondence, and reporting.

Policies and procedures are also important elements for HRPP accreditation and for the institution's reputation. Standards for accreditation often request information about audit procedures, compliance, and quality assessment/improvement. For example, Alion Science and Technology provides HRPP accreditation services and requires that "the organization has policies, procedures and practices for monitoring and auditing functions of the IRB and other organizational entities to ensure compliance and promote quality assessment and improvement" (Standard 11).[1] Additionally, AAHRPP accreditation standards require that, "[t]he Organization measures and improves, when necessary, compliance with organizational policies and procedures and applicable laws, regulations, codes, and guidance [. . . as well as] the quality, effectiveness, and efficiency of the Human Research Protection Program" (Standard I-5).[2] The existence of, and compliance with, policies further help to protect the reputation of the organization if—and when—an untoward event occurs.

Table 3.3. Descriptions of institutional documents related to IRBs and QA/QI programs

Document Type	Description
IRB Policy	Establishes IRB in compliance with law and regulations and sets forth requirements for IRB review of all human subject research conducted in the institution; establishes IRB authority and limits thereof; may delineate responsibilities for written procedures or alternative approaches
IRB Procedures	Procedures detailing every facet of IRB establishment, operations, and oversight; roles and responsibilities of institution and institutional official, IRB administrative staff, IRB members, investigators, sponsors, and others; reporting requirements; etc.
QA/QI Policy	Institutional policy for QA/QI program (scope and responsibility for assuring compliance); procedures for assuring IRB, investigators, and staff are in compliance

Policies and Procedures for Other Programs within an HRPP

Another fundamental role of a QA/QI program is to assure institutional leadership that each department comprising the HRPP is in compliance with institutional and, when applicable, departmental policies and procedures. Thus, when conducting a review or audit, a QA/QI reviewer should first identify the policies and procedures that apply to the group and the activity. The QA/QI reviewer should then evaluate the policies and procedures themselves to ensure that each document is clear, includes all the elements, meets institutional expectations (i.e., identify any gaps or overlaps with other groups), and incorporates applicable federal and state laws and regulations. See Table 3.3 for descriptions of different institutional documents related to IRB and QA/QI programs.

Whenever an institutional or departmental policy or procedure is reviewed, we recommend that the reviewer attend to its clarity and completeness. If a member of the QA/QI program finds either a policy or procedure confusing or unclear, others will have similar difficulty. Constructive suggestions for improvement should be brought to the manager or director of the program, and if sufficiently serious, follow-up should be expected.

Points to Consider
Audience
Every policy and procedures document should have a defined audience; the audience may impact the style and tone of the document, as well as the degree of specificity required. When specifying the responsible par-

ties, use job titles (e.g., institutional official (IO), IRB chair) and not the specific names of the individuals currently occupying the positions. If the policy or procedure directs communication or responsibility to a specific recipient, consider creating a generic e-mail address specific to the issue (e.g., SAEreport@institution.org) or the individual (IRBchair@institution .org). Rendering the position as a generic function, independent of the individual currently holding the position, will limit revisions to the policy for trivial rather than substantive changes. Any such mailbox must be monitored regularly as an assigned job responsibility.

Policy Scope

Policies and procedures are the strategic link between the vision of a QA/QI program and its activities and daily operations. QA/QI policies should be envisioned and written with careful consideration of practices, performance expectations, and compliance. External auditors monitor compliance with laws and regulations and institutional policies and procedures; if the expectations of the institutional policy exceed the law or regulation, institutions—and their leaders and staff—must comply with the higher standard. Policies that raise the standards above OHRP, FDA, Office of Civil Rights, and other applicable regulations, therefore, deserve special consideration.

Institutional Consistency and Integration

Institutional policies should be consistent with and complement one another. For example, the policy of the QA/QI program cannot conflict with other, relevant institutional policies (e.g., IRB, research compliance). If, for example, an IRB policy requires serious adverse event (SAE) reporting within 72 hours, the QA/QI program policy should not give a different time window, and preferably would write its own policy in reference to that of the IRB (e.g., "QA/QI should monitor adverse event reports to determine that reporting is complete within the time course specified by the IRB"). It is advisable, therefore, to share draft policies widely and solicit feedback specifically from individuals and offices with whom interaction is likely.

Institutional Support

All institutional policies should be supported by leadership and have the resources necessary for enforcement. Institutional committees, the HRPP director, IRB chair(s), the IO, general counsel, and/or compliance offices should be involved in reviewing policies before they are finalized and communicated and as they are updated. The appropriate institutional authorities should review and approve each policy and update prior to dissemination.

Accessibility

Policies and procedures are only as useful as they are accessible to the intended audience. Transparency and broad communication of QA/QI policies to the research community is an important early step in implementation. The avenues of dissemination (e.g., website, newsletters) of a new, revised, or updated policy should be planned in advance of its effective date but merely communicating the availability of a new or updated policy is insufficient. Periodic education and reminders may be necessary for current staff, and newly employed staff should be trained appropriately. All policies and procedures should be accessible on a common website that is known to the affected audience.

Training

Communication regarding a policy must be complemented with training and education on the policy itself, including its specific expectations and intended application. Training is an important means of ensuring the affected audience(s) understands the policy's implications and anticipated procedures, which will ultimately help promote compliance. When planning educational programming, the choice of format (e.g., e-mail notice, in-person educational sessions, online courses) and method of documentation ("I have read and understand . . .") is likely to vary based on the policy and the audience.

Services, Guides, and Tools

Institutions can and should develop services, guides, and tools to help researchers, study teams, and staff execute planned research activities with integrity and in compliance with local, state, and federal laws and regulations and institutional policies and procedures. Investigators and their research staff should be strongly encouraged to access these services and use or adapt these documents to manage their research.

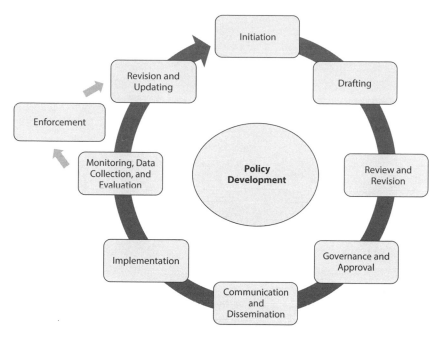

Figure 3.2. Policy Development Cycle

Continuous Learning

An advantage of utilizing forms and checklists for QA/QI activities, including monitoring and audits, is the standardization of data collection. The QA/QI program should aggregate and analyze its own data with some periodicity, and not less than annually, to determine if there are systemic deficiencies, opportunities, or strengths. We recommend this exercise be formalized into an annual report that includes an overview of the QA/QI program's work and its findings, analysis, and recommendations for future activities (Figure 3.2).

SUMMARY

- Policies describe *what* the policy is and *why* it should be followed.

- Procedures describe *how* and *when* to use the policy and *who* should follow it.

- Policies and procedures can facilitate consistency, build trust, foster transparency, and serve as an effective method of documenting processes.

- Evaluate policies and procedures for clarity and completeness; ensure they include applicable institutional, local, and federal expectations and regulations.

- Consider your audience, scope, and support of the institution when creating procedures and policies.

REFERENCES

1. Alion Science and Technology, "Alion HRPP Accreditation Standards."

2. Association for the Accreditation of Human Research Protection Programs, Inc., "Domain I: Organization."

4

Investigator Site Review

Susan Corl, Alyssa Gateman, Nareg D. Grigorian, and Sarah A. White

Purpose

A foundational activity of any QA/QI program or function is an internal evaluation of investigator compliance. This evaluation is often referred to as an "investigator site review" but may also be referred to as a "study visit," "study review," "study audit," "internal audit," or "educational audit."

The primary goal of an investigator site review is to assess study-specific compliance with applicable requirements governing human subjects' protection, including (1) federal regulations,[1] (2) local institutional policies and/or guidelines, and (3) good clinical practice (GCP). The review process provides an opportunity for real time, one-on-one training and education of investigator(s) and the research team. This chapter describes the different types, as well as the components, of an investigator site review.

Types and Triggers

There are two general types of investigator site reviews: *routine* and *directed*. Routine, or not-for-cause, investigator site reviews may be initiated as part of an overall institutional strategy (e.g., QA/QI-initiated or at random) or initiated at the request of the principal investigator (PI) and study staff. Routine reviews serve as a prospective method of assessing compliance and adherence to requirements. They can and should be conducted early in the active phase of participant enrollment and data collection (e.g., after the third participant is enrolled) in order to identify areas of noncompliance early. Directed, or for-cause, site reviews are initiated

Table 4.1. Possible triggers for routine and directed investigator site reviews

Type of investigator site review	Possible triggers
Routine	• Institutional goal (e.g., to conduct site reviews for a certain percentage of overall research portfolio within a given time period) • Institutional policy (e.g., to conduct routine reviews for a "first-time" Principal Investigator (PI); student researchers; off-campus research; or multicenter, PI-initiated trials) • Investigator/site initiated (e.g., when there is a new study PI, study personnel turnover, or self-identified noncompliance; in anticipation of an anticipated external audit (e.g., FDA audit); for study close-out; or for educational purposes)
Directed	• Identified need for education / record keeping (i.e., to ensure adequate study documentation and understanding of applicable regulations, institutional policies, and GCP) • IRB-suspected noncompliance based on observations by IRB administrator or convened IRB • Self-report of possible serious or continuing noncompliance • Report of noncompliance from a third party

based on concerns (suspected, reported, or documented), complaints, or allegations of noncompliance raised by a study participant, an IRB, the study sponsor, or a federal agency charged with oversight of clinical research (e.g., FDA). A directed review can be conducted on behalf of an IRB, IO, or other designated HRPP official. Examples of possible triggers for routine and directed site reviews can be found in Table 4.1.

Process

The investigator site review process includes not only the discrete time scheduled at the investigator's site but also the process of determining the scope of the review, and the time required for site notification, QA/QI reviewer preparation, drafting of the written report, and post-review education, if necessary (Figure 4.1). The reviewer(s) should work with the investigator(s) and their research team to ensure that all parties have a clear understanding of the totality of the review process.

Determining Scope of Review

A QA/QI program may develop some general core criteria that all investigator site reviews will cover. These may include review of PI delegation, training, informed consent documents, and participant files. How-

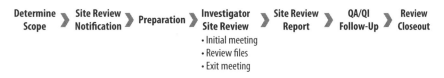

Determine Scope › Site Review Notification › Preparation › Investigator Site Review • Initial meeting • Review files • Exit meeting › Site Review Report › QA/QI Follow-Up › Review Closeout

Figure 4.1. Investigator site review process

ever, each investigator site review should also develop a specific and defined scope for each site review and this will direct the QA/QI reviewers in their preparation and execution of the site review. The following six elements may determine the scope of the review:

1. Type of review
2. Purpose/trigger of the review
3. Study status
4. Total number of enrolled subjects
5. Identified noncompliance, if any
6. Available QA/QI resources

Prior to arriving on site, the QA/QI program (or other appropriate body) should communicate the scope of the site review to the investigator and research team. When a study has been active for many years (e.g., spanning from paper to electronic records and/or over a time period during which policies and practices have changed significantly), the scope of the site review may be limited to a defined period of time (e.g., last three years). Additionally, if appropriate, the investigator may assist in directing the scope of the review by identifying areas of concern.

Investigator Site Review Notification to Investigator and Research Team

The key to a successful review is to establish and maintain clear and open lines of communication between the investigators, the research team, and those performing the site review. Depending on the site review type and trigger, notification may be made by an IO, the IRB, or the QA/QI program. The following information should be provided in the notification, which can be sent to the PI via e-mail:

- Study to be reviewed (official title, protocol #, and IRB #, if available).
- Purpose of the site review.

- Information to be reviewed (e.g., regulatory binder, consent forms, participant files).
- Who is required to be at the site review (e.g., the investigator and key members of the study team must be available for the initial and exit meetings/interviews. Note: each institution/program will need to determine the details of these requirements).
- An agenda (including kickoff meeting, review of documents, and exit meeting) and approximate amount of time needed for the review.
- Time frame during which the site review will be conducted (Note: often it is more efficient and respectful for the QA/QI program to suggest several possible dates and times from which the investigator may choose).
- Access requirements and the need for physical and/or electronic access to facilities and electronic data capture systems (Note: This should be determined and provided for prior to the reviewer's arrival on site).

Preparation for Site Review

The QA/QI reviewer(s) should be well prepared prior to arriving on site. Depending on the QA/QI program structure and available resources, a decision should be made regarding how many QA/QI reviewers will conduct the on-site review. The reviewer(s) should be familiar with the following information:

- Protocol
- Applicable regulatory and policy requirements
- PI delegation to study team
- Number of participants enrolled to date
- IRB correspondence to date (including reported events, protocol amendments, changes to consent forms, etc.)
- How the site has documented the study (e.g., paper files, electronic files, or a combination of both)

The QA/QI reviewer(s) should gather enough information ahead of time to ensure access to, and familiarity with, the systems necessary to conduct a useful review. For example, knowledge of previously reported protocol noncompliance can be ascertained via IRB records in preparation for the site review. A coded enrollment log can be requested in advance to understand the number and status of enrolled participants.

The QA/QI reviewer(s) should decide whether the investigator will be told in advance what specific records are to be reviewed. The decision as to whether or not to inform the investigator may depend on the impetus for the review and the type of review being conducted. Wherein the review is meant to assess actual practices, it may be useful—and more helpful to the investigator and their study team—to perform the review without the time for the site to prepare. If long lead times are given, and specific information is provided about the scope of record review, well-meaning research team members may concentrate efforts and focus on the specified study records in preparation for the review and may do so with a narrowed focus and without best practices in mind, leaving other records untouched, and as a result, possibly noncompliant.

If the IRB of record is local to the site, a complete IRB review history should be available to the QA/QI reviewer. If the IRB of record is not local, only a more limited review history may be available. IRB records may be paper, electronic, or a combination of both. QA/QI programs should be able to access paper files or have electronic access for all studies. Depending on the scope of the review, it may be appropriate for the QA/QI reviewer to also review records from other offices or entities, including: clinical trials office, grants and contracts, radiation/biosafety, conflict of interest committee, HIPAA/privacy board, ClinicalTrials.gov database, etc.

Typically, QA/QI programs develop evaluation tools to conduct a review. The evaluation tool should enable the QA/QI reviewer to document in detail any noncompliance found during the on-site review. The evaluation tool may contain a core set of criteria that allows for consistent assessments to be made across all types of audits and research protocols, for example: PI delegation, documentation of informed consent, COI disclosure/reporting, data security practices, etc. An example of a comprehensive evaluation tool (titled "Model Audit Tool") can be found in Appendix B.

The evaluation tool may also contain initial meeting and/or exit meeting questions. Site practice and protocol-specific questions enable the QA/QI reviewers to understand the study's progress from the investigator and/or study team perspective. Interview questions may also identify noncompliance that may not be easy to identify in the documented materials. For instance, a reviewer may ask whether any participants enrolled were non-English speaking, and if so, how they provided their informed consent.

It is essential for QA/QI reviewers to document specific observations while also protecting the private information of participants. A QA/QI reviewer may document participant ID, date of visit, or other information that may identify the participants; however, the reviewer should take steps to minimize the collection of information that could directly identify participants and should store all data according to the institution's policies and practices.

Investigator Site Review

A typical investigator site review has three components: the initial meeting, the review of study files, and the exit interview.

INITIAL MEETING

Investigators and study teams may feel intimidated or threatened by an on-site review, especially a review that is conducted for-cause. An initial meeting, during which expectations are set and questions answered, may help reduce anxiety. Generally speaking, audits are intended to assist the investigator in producing high-quality research and ensure participant safety. Establishing a collegial, consultative tone can set the stage for a successful review. The QA/QI reviewer(s) should ask the research team to designate a team member who will be available throughout the review process to address any questions that may arise. During this initial meeting, the reviewer(s) should also inform the investigator and study team that they will be kept abreast of findings as the review unfolds, which will reduce the likelihood of the team receiving "surprise findings" at the end of the review process.

REVIEW OF STUDY FILES

The review of study files is generally conducted without the investigator or study staff present in order to have an undirected, objective review of the accuracy and completeness of the files. If investigators and study staff are present, they may be inclined to direct and/or interpret study documentation for the QA/QI reviewer.

Depending on the capacity of the QA/QI program, reviewers may have limited time and resources to commit to reviews. As such, a QA/QI program should consider time management and effectiveness strategies in the records-review process and whether all or only a sample of study files are reviewed.

Depending on the purpose of the site review and QA/QI program resources, all or some of the following areas may be reviewed:

- Regulatory documentation / study management tools
- Subject informed consent
- Subject eligibility information
- Protocol adherence
- Drug/device accountability

Table 4.2 provides details and examples of each category of documentation that maybe be reviewed and specific examples.

A number of different considerations determine the sample size of the site review, as shown schematically in Figure 4.2. The QA/QI reviewer may review 100 percent of the study files or choose a sample of study files, and the file sample may be chosen by either a random or nonrandom selection. When a random sample of study files will be selected, the QA/QI program can use a random number generator. The random numbers are matched to a study subject ID or place in enrollment. If a nonrandom sample of study files will be selected, the reviewer will pick and choose which files to audit. This may happen because the reviewer has information that would lead to review of a particular set of subject files (e.g., all study participants who underwent a certain research procedure or study participants that were consented by a particular investigator). Again, it is important that the reviewer collects the minimal amount of information to avoid enabling the direct identification of study participants.

EXIT MEETING AND REVIEW OF FINDINGS

The exit meeting is conducted for the purpose of conveying the reviewer's preliminary findings to the investigator / study staff and to address any issues that can be resolved at that time. The QA/QI program should specify who should be present at the exit meeting. The meeting should be held in a private location and include a summary of all the observations that the reviewer has made with respect to overall study compliance. QA/QI reviewers should provide the regulatory context for, and specific details

Table 4.2. Categories and examples of study documentation that may be reviewed during an audit

Review category	Study documentation*
Regulatory documentation / study management tools	• Enrollment log • Delegation of responsibility • Staff qualifications (CV, medical/clinical licensure) • Laboratory certification and normal value ranges • Sponsor correspondence • IRB documentation (all significant correspondence submitted to or received from the IRB, including submissions, investigator responses, notification letters, and approved consent forms) • Documentation of data and safety monitoring, including log of monitoring activities, meeting agendas, minutes and reports of the data monitoring committee
Subject informed consent	• Informed consent document • Documentation of informed consent • Re-consent, if required
Subject eligibility information	• Source documentation verifying inclusion and exclusion criteria according to IRB-approved protocol (e.g., screening form, intake questionnaire, medical record information, self-report)
Protocol adherence	• Study procedures according to IRB-approved protocol • Pretreatment/therapy requirements • Follow-up visits/communications • Treatment administration and dose modifications • Adverse events • Unanticipated events • Protocol deviations and exceptions (e.g., one-time modifications)
Drug/device accountability	• Receipt of drug/device • Storage conditions • Administration/implant • Disposal (including destruction of expired product)
Data security	• Data security provisions implemented to protect confidentiality
Subject payment records	• Payment receipts • Payment or reimbursement logs
Grant/funding documentation	• Grant (salaries may be redacted) or attestation that there has not been a change to the grant or a progress report • OHRP declaration of assurance of the grant • Sponsor correspondence

*These are examples; this is not intended to serve as an exhaustive listing.

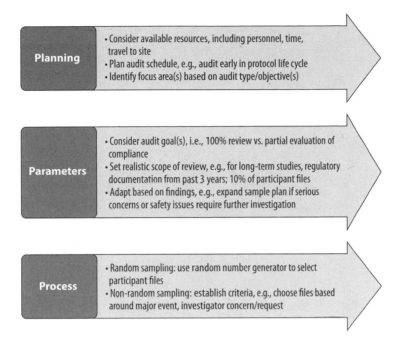

Figure 4.2. Identifying sample size for review

of, the observations, citing the specific regulation, policy, or other source, if possible.

The exit meeting also provides an opportunity to discuss any questions related to the findings, the conduct of the study, and overall best practices, as well as any corrective actions that the investigator and study team can or must make to improve study conduct and facilitate compliance. During the meeting, the QA/QI reviewer should also go over the process for reviewing the investigator site review report (see description below), including when the investigator will receive the report, who will have access to it, how it will be used, and what responsibilities the investigator has after receiving the report. The exit meeting is a very useful educational opportunity and should be explicitly framed as such.

Report

The QA/QI program should provide the investigator with a comprehensive report summarizing the site review and memorializing any

Table 4.3. Suggested elements to include in an investigator site review report

Suggested element	Suggested details
Cover page	• Protocol • Investigator name • Date of review • Date of report • QA/QI reviewer(s)
Introduction	• Purpose of site review • Individuals present at meeting • Material reviewed at the time of site review (e.g., regulatory documentation, all consent forms, and subject files for XX of YY subjects)
Observations	• Provide specific examples and sufficient detail so that site can identify individual errors (see "Observation Index" below) • Consider providing regulatory references and corrective actions (see "Regulatory References" below)
Conclusion	• Summarize the site review and provide contact for questions • Consider identifying priorities for the site (see "Identifying Priorities" below) • Consider "grading" the report (see "'Grading' the Report" below) • If response from site is required, identify timeline for response (see "Corrective and Preventive Action" below)

observations that were made, including any specific problems. Overall, site review reports should be concise, objective, and easy for the investigator and study staff to understand. Use tables and bullets rather than long narratives. The QA/QI reviewer(s) should provide the report to the investigator in a timely fashion, generally within two weeks of the exit meeting. Table 4.3 includes suggested elements in an investigative site review report.

Additional Report Considerations

- *Regulatory References.* Investigators and study staff may not be familiar with the specific applicable regulations and/or institutional policies that are required for human research. Therefore, it is helpful for the QA/QI program to identify the associated regulatory reference for each observation in the report.
- *Corrective and Preventive Actions.* Generally, reports provide specific, instructive corrective actions for each observation or general best

practice recommendations or request that the investigator develop his/her own corrective action plan. If providing a corrective action for each observation in the report, the program should clearly communicate the steps required to achieve the corrective action (e.g., report to the IRB as a violation or write a note-to-file) and provide links to tools or checklists to aid/educate the investigator and study staff. If an investigator is responsible for developing a corrective action plan, the program should assist the investigator by providing applicable policies and/or educational tools.

- *Identifying Priorities.* In some cases, the site review may reveal numerous observations spanning different areas of research practice and documentation. Providing a report with twenty-plus observations can be overwhelming to investigators. In these cases, consider identifying priorities for the site to focus on, identifying the set of related observations, and providing steps to achieving compliance in these areas.

- *Observation Index.* Regardless of the number of full-time employees, a QA/QI program must address the consistency, and subsequent communication, of their observations. Many established programs have managed this by creating a standardized set or list of observations (Table 4.4). A standardized set of observations should cover any observation that can be made, categorized by topic and associated with regulatory references and corrective actions. New observations can and should be added to the list as needed. Details of the study-specific observations should accompany the standardized observation in the investigator site review report. An example of an expanded observation index can be found in the Appendix B.

- *Standardized Categories of Noncompliance.* In order to recognize that observations of noncompliance are of varying severity and consequence, the QA/QI program may wish to establish and define categories to assign to each observation (e.g., major noncompliance, minor noncompliance, noncompliance with GCP or record keeping guidelines). This categorization assists in measuring overall noncompliance and in analysis of aggregate data (see Chapter 6). The QA/QI program may wish to maintain this categorization for internal communication only (e.g., IRB, research compliance, office of

Table 4.4. Select examples of standardized general and specific observations

General observation(s)	Additional specific details provided in report
Study procedures were performed by individuals who lack IRB approval.	• Subjects A1, B2, and C3 were consented by an attending physician not listed in the IRB-approved protocol.
Changes were made to study procedures without IRB approval.	• Surrogate consent was obtained for subjects A1 and B2. The IRB has not approved a surrogate consent process for this study.
Copy of education certificate and completed study-specific trainings for all members of the study team are not on file.	• Current human research training documentation, as well as study-specific trainings, are not on file for the co-investigator and RA. Research education certificate expired for the research coordinator.
Errors in records corrected with scribble over incorrect information.	• Observed instances of errors scribbled over as method of correction in subject files A1, B2, and C3. Research data and records should be attributable, legible, contemporaneous, original, accurate ("ALCOA"). Errors should be corrected with a single strike / horizontal line through the incorrect information and insertion of the correct information; the correction should be initialed/signed and dated. Do not erase, scribble out/over, or use correction fluid or any other means that could obscure original entry/information.
Data collection form not completed.	• Questionnaire and participant assessment for subject G7 incomplete. Note: This missing document serves as source documentation for case report forms. Missing data may have implications for the scientific integrity of the study.
Informed consent form not properly completed.	• Signature of investigator and printed investigator name not completed (page 12 of ICF) for subject D4.
Deviations from IRB-approved protocol.	• Subject A1: Visits occurred outside of ± 7-day window. Appears subject should have already undergone Visit 3 by 03/07/2015 (6 months, ± 7 days); no data on file. • Subject B2: Visit 1 05/03/2019, Visit 2 (3 months, ± 7 days) occurred on 08/25/2019.
Content on ClinicalTrials.gov not current.	• This is an applicable clinical trial; website information is to be updated at least every 12 months. Review requirements associated with registration; periodically monitor/review information on www.clinicaltrials.gov, and update current website posting.

general counsel, institutional leadership) versus sharing with investigators and study staff. Before finalizing the categories, the groups receiving the information should provide input. The content should strive to be helpful to the investigators and their research teams as well as the recipients.

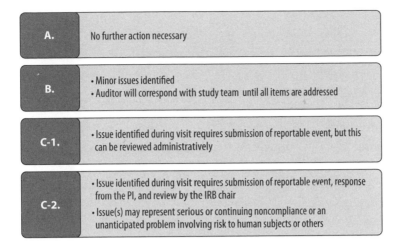

A.	No further action necessary
B.	• Minor issues identified • Auditor will correspond with study team until all items are addressed
C-1.	• Issue identified during visit requires submission of reportable event, but this can be reviewed administratively
C-2.	• Issue identified during visit requires submission of reportable event, response from the PI, and review by the IRB chair • Issue(s) may represent serious or continuing noncompliance or an unanticipated problem involving risk to human subjects or others

Figure 4.3. Example of QA/QI Report Grading System. Used by permission of University of Pittsburgh, Education and Compliance Office for Human Subject Research

- *"Grading" the Report.* QA/QI programs may wish to "grade" or categorize reports (Figure 4.3). Grading reports can serve as a tool to communicate to the investigator and/or other institutional representatives how well the overall study is being conducted and the severity of the problems identified. When developing a grading scale, a QA/QI program should seek input and agreement from relevant institutional stakeholders including IOs, the office of general counsel, IRB committees, and investigators.

- *Internal Committee to Review Reports.* An institution may decide that an internal oversight committee may review some or all QA/QI reports. Generally, the oversight committee will review the final report, may "grade" the report, categorize the findings, and/or request additional follow-up information, a corrective action plan, and/or response to the report. The process and function of this committee should be clearly outlined in QA/QI standard operating procedures and institutional policies and procedures.

- *Report Access.* It is important to consider who will receive, and have access to, the report. In all cases, the investigator and study team should have access. In some institutions, the IRB may also have access to reports, while other institutions may provide the reports to the IRB only when the review is requested by the IRB. Generally, the reports are not given to an industry or government (e.g., NIH) sponsor, external monitor, or regulatory agency such as OHRP or the FDA. Instead, if requested, a summary of the observations can be provided to these external parties. The provision of a site review certificate may provide an alternative to providing a summary; this certificate does not typically specify any observations or outcome of the site review but is a confirmation that a site review took place. It is strongly encouraged that an institution's office of general counsel be consulted regarding who has access to QA/QI program reports and how to maintain confidentiality of the findings, if appropriate.

QA/QI Follow-Up

When considering the type of follow-up, if any, for each investigator site review, the QA/QI program should consider three factors:

1. Type of noncompliance found during the site review
2. Level of investigator/staff knowledge regarding research requirements
3. Capacity of the QA/QI program to provide follow-up support

Follow-up actions may include

- Documentation of findings and discrepancy(ies) (e.g., writing a note-to-file)
- Mandatory training/retraining of investigator and/or study team
- Reporting noncompliance to the IRB
- Additional reviews of the same study at a later date
- Reviews of all the investigator's studies
- Assigned mentorship

Additionally, the QA/QI program may assist the PI / study team in implementing corrective actions / best practice recommendations (Figure 4.4). Individual reviewers may be assigned to evaluate and/or follow-up on investigator responses and corrective actions. QA/QI managers may take on these responsibilities or formal institutional oversight committees may be formed, the latter of which is particularly appropriate when serious or continuing noncompliance is observed.

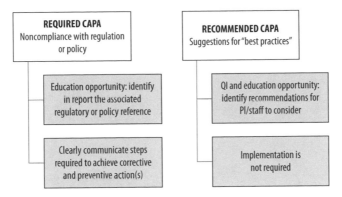

Figure 4.4. Required vs. recommended corrective and preventive actions (CAPA)

Review Closeout

The QA/QI program should consider developing a formal process for closing out the review. The closeout communication summary should include three points:

1. Dates of the review
2. Final determination, if categorized and/or graded
3. Follow-up, if applicable

Notification of closeout can be as simple as an e-mail to the investigator and study team, documenting that the process is complete, or a more formal, standardized memo template. At the conclusion of an investigator site review, it is natural for a QA/QI program to consider how the overall process could be improved. This can be accomplished by inviting participating investigators and study staff to complete a formal evaluation or, more simply, to address a few questions most relevant to the QA/QI program about the review process. In addition, a QA/QI program may wish to retain and analyze investigator site review findings as a means to identify systematic compliance issues and prevent future reoccurrence. Analyzing aggregate data can better inform and focus a QA/QI program's education and training efforts as well as the study management tools they choose to develop and refine. For further discussion, see Chapter 6.

SUMMARY

- There are two general types of investigator site reviews—*routine* and *directed*.

- Routine (also called "not-for-cause") site reviews may be initiated as part of overall institutional strategy or initiated at the request of the PI/study staff.

- Directed (also called "for-cause") site reviews are initiated based on concerns, complaints, or allegations of noncompliance raised by a study participant, an IRB, the study sponsor, or a federal agency charged with oversight of clinical research.

- The investigator site review process consists of the following steps: determine scope, notify site of review, prepare for the review, conduct investigator site review, create site review report, follow-up, review closeout.

- QA/QI programs should consider how the overall investigator site review process could be improved, seeking input from investigators and study staff and/or analyzing reviewing findings to identify compliance issues and prevent future reoccurrences.

REFERENCE

1. US Food and Drug Administration, "E6(R2) Good Clinical Practice: Integrated Addendum to ICH E6(R1) Guidance for Industry."

5

Evaluating IRB Compliance

Jennifer A. Graf, Leslie M. Howes, Cynthia Monahan,
Eunice Newbert, and Sarah A. White

Purpose

Conducting an investigator site review to evaluate and facilitate investigator compliance is a hallmark of any QA/QI program. QA/QI programs can provide similar proactive services to the IRB, perform periodic evaluation of IRB files, and make recommendations to improve the overall conduct, efficiency, and compliance of IRB functions.

The purpose of an IRB evaluation is to assess IRB compliance with applicable regulations, institutional policies, and good clinical practice guidelines. The QA/QI program does not review the ethical discussions of any protocol or any IRB board meeting, nor does it review decisions made by the IRB but rather focuses upon the operations, efficiency, and compliance of the IRB office. Similar to investigator site reviews, an inspection or review of IRB files provides an opportunity to identify common issues, harmonize and/or strengthen practices, improve efficiency and accuracy, provide feedback and education to IRB reviewers and staff, prevent IRB noncompliance, and evaluate the larger HRPP. The findings are also often helpful to institutional leadership.

This chapter provides an introduction to some QA/QI activities designed to evaluate IRB compliance, including reviews of IRB files, meeting minutes, and membership composition.

IRB File Review

The framework below outlines how a QA/QI program may implement IRB file review as a standalone activity and/or as a precursor to and in conjunction with an investigator site review. Specifically, this section addresses potential triggers that may prompt the review of IRB files and who may be best suited to conduct such a review. In addition, this section provides a discussion of the mechanics involved in IRB file review, which include consideration for periodicity, access, scope, and content.

When to Conduct a Review of IRB Files

A number of circumstances may prompt a review of IRB files. Conducting such a review can occur as a complement to investigator site reviews (referred to as a "360°" review) or independently of them (Figure 5.1).

- *Complementary IRB File Review.* Quite often, an IRB file review occurs as a natural complement to the customary directed (for-cause) and/or routine (not-for-cause) investigator site reviews. These reviews include examination of study documentation maintained by both the IRB and the investigator, thereby providing a more complete evaluation of compliance than looking at each independently. Further, evaluating IRB files can foster a greater sense of transparency and goodwill among the research community by holding the IRB accountable for its own actions and demonstrating the independence of the QA/QI program from the IRB. The latter is significant when the organizational structure does not clearly delineate between IRB and QA/QI operations, as discussed in Chapter 2 of this handbook. When conducting a complementary IRB file review, any report of findings should be directed to the IRB and not to the investigator and study staff.
- *Independent IRB File Review.* An IRB file review conducted independently from an investigator site review can provide significant benefit on its own. Such review may be conducted at regular intervals as a means of evaluating and improving IRB compliance and best practices. Alternatively, when resources are limited, a program may conduct such reviews only as needed or in direct response to reported or alleged noncompliance, an anticipated external inspection by the FDA, a sponsor, or an accreditation site visit (e.g., AAHRPP).

Considerations for IRB File Selection

Several factors may influence how a program selects files for an IRB file review (Figure 5.2).

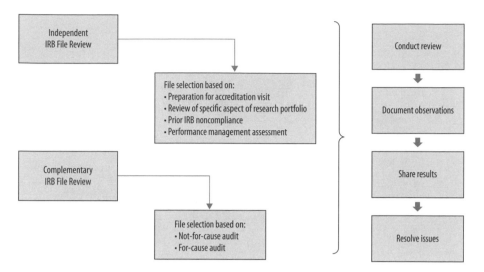

Figure 5.1. Flowchart for independent and complementary IRB file review

- *Institutional Considerations.* Program leadership should consider whether an IRB file review may be helpful in furthering institutional strategies or compliance with HRPP policies. For example, if the institution is preparing for accreditation and/or external inspection, the program may wish to focus on review of the IRB files likely to be audited by the external site visitors/inspectors. Alternatively, the implementation of a new or a revised policy or practice may help to identify a group of files related to the practice or policy appropriate for review.
- *Research Portfolio.* It may be helpful to identify unique aspects of an institution's research portfolio. For instance, if the portfolio is primarily social-behavioral-education research, a review of biomedical studies may be valuable, as the IRB's review experience in this area may be limited. Alternatively, a program may consider a risk-based approach by focusing on protocols posing greater than minimal risk, protocols involving new research methodologies or investigational products, or protocols with numerous amendment requests. If the sample requires further filtering, focusing on a specific protocol type, (e.g., sponsor-investigator IND/IDE studies) or a particular determination (e.g., inclusion of vulnerable population) may be helpful.

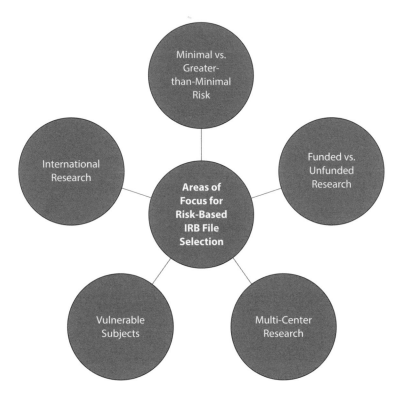

Figure 5.2. Risk-based considerations for IRB file selection

- *Prior Noncompliance.* Prior IRB noncompliance may also influence IRB file review selection. In revisiting such cases, a program can determine whether corrective actions and/or best practice recommendations have been understood, implemented, and sustained. If noncompliance persists, such a review provides an opportunity for improvement through additional IRB member training or the development or revision of IRB reviewer tools, IRB staff retraining, etc.
- *Performance Management.* Although many institutions rely on the human resources department to structure the criteria for performance review, this process may not sufficiently highlight competencies particularly relevant and unique to the function and operations of an IRB. When considering performance management, an IRB staff member's supervisor or the collective QA/QI group might review a sample of IRB files to reveal areas of weakness that could benefit

Table 5.1. Information evaluated as part of an IRB file review and sources for that information

Information to review	Source of information
Description of the proposed study	• Original and revised IRB applications/forms, protocol, recruitment and consent materials, study tools, cede review plans, IRB meeting minutes, etc.
Documentation of IRB review and determination(s)	• IRB reviewer checklists, worksheets, and notes; IRB meeting minutes; formal IRB correspondence to the PI
IRB notification letter(s)	• IRB correspondence sent to the PI outlining a determination and/or decision (e.g., approval letter)
Significant correspondence	• Letters, e-mails, or documented telephone calls that contribute to the IRB's overall analysis of the proposed study; communication and documentation related to IRB authorization requests; COI-related information
Applicable external/ ancillary review(s)	• Documentation of review and/or approval from external groups, as appropriate (e.g., institution biosafety committee, embryonic stem cell research oversight committee, radiation safety committee, investigational drug service, scientific review committee, outside consultants)

from additional training or to highlight potential best practices and models for others in the office.

Table 5.1 describes information that maybe be evaluated during an IRB file review and sources for that information.

Mechanics of an IRB File Review

When preparing to conduct an IRB file review, consider several logistics, including periodicity, access, scope, and content.

- *Periodicity*. Programs should determine when an IRB file review should occur. This may be as simple as implementing a policy establishing a 360° review and requiring the IRB file review as a preliminary step for any investigator site review (directed or routine). Alternatively, programs may elect to conduct an IRB file review as a standalone compliance activity on a monthly or quarterly basis, or simply as needed.
- *Access*. A QA/QI reviewer should be familiar with the IRB's submission formatting. Some IRBs rely solely on paper-based methods,

others use electronic submission capture, while some use a combination of both. Further still, electronic submission platforms differ significantly. For instance, some systems completely automate the submission process, including workflow support, while others serve as an electronic repository of uploaded documents. The QA/QI reviewer must be able to access all protocol documentation, regardless of the format in which it is stored.

- *Scope.* A complete file review is the gold standard; however, the review scope may need to be reduced depending on both the scale of the study and the available resources for the review. If scope must be narrowed, partial reviews may include (a) reviewing documentation since the last continuing review or (b) focusing the review on an area of concern or prior compliance issue (e.g., ensuring proper documentation is on file and requisite IRB findings are documented supporting the inclusion of a vulnerable population). Be mindful of how scope may change depending on the trigger for a review. A routine IRB file review, for example, may not warrant an evaluation of all available documentation (unless something that requires follow-up and further investigation is found), whereas a directed (for-cause) review may initially focus on an area of concern and then expand until all relevant documentation has been evaluated.

- *Content.* The review is likely to include documentation of IRB reviews, determinations, and notification letters, as well as significant correspondence between the IRB and PI or others including federal regulators, sponsors, and/or the funding agency/ies, as appropriate. Such documentation is customarily stored in a single location, such as a protocol-specific file; however, additional documentation that can serve to validate, or possibly refute, a QA/QI reviewer's observations may exist elsewhere. For example, review of the IRB meeting minutes would serve to verify determinations and requests for information, amendments, and/or revisions.

Table 5.2 depicts examples of findings from audits of IRB files.

IRB Meeting Minutes Review

Federal regulations require that an institution or IRB prepare and maintain adequate documentation of IRB activities, including minutes of

Table 5.2. Examples of common findings from audit of IRB files

Common findings	Applicable Regulations
Not all IRB documentation is found on file (e.g., current protocol/ ICF/assent form; COI disclosure forms; copy of signed IRB-approved letter to PI; local ethical approval).	45 CFR 46.115(a)(1)* 21 CFR 56.115(a)(1)**
Documentation of correspondence between the IRB and investigators is not found on file (e.g., e-mails not in file, note-to-file re: telephone or in-person conversation missing).	21 CFR 56.115(a)(4)**
Findings not documented for new minimal risk studies and/or expedited continuing review and/or amendments.	45 CFR 46.109(e)*
IRB approval for the study lapsed; documentation alerting the PI is not on file.	45 CFR 46.108(a)(3)(i)* 21 CFR 56.108(a)(1)**
The electronically submitted documents sent by the PI are not signed.	N/A

*Office for Human Research Protections, "45 CFR 46 Protection of Human Subjects."
**US Food and Drug Administration, "21 CFR 56 FDA Regulations Institutional Review Boards."

IRB meetings. Although the regulations specify certain required content,[1] the approach and format for documenting them frequently vary, depending on an IRB's policies, procedures, and practices. As such, a QA/QI program should be well versed in institutional policies and procedures with respect to IRB meeting conduct, including its template for meeting minutes. Indeed, review of the template itself is a valuable activity.

Considerations for IRB Meeting Minutes Review

Although many of the considerations raised above relating to the mechanics of IRB file review also apply to the review of IRB meeting minutes, the following points highlight some areas requiring further consideration.

- *Periodicity*. A program should consider the convened IRB meeting schedule when determining the appropriate frequency to review meeting minutes. For instance, if the convened IRB meets monthly, a program may choose to review meeting minutes on a monthly schedule as well. If the convened IRB meets weekly, a program may review minutes on a weekly basis or may instead choose to conduct such a review on a monthly basis for some or all meetings within that month. When possible, the IRB should not be aware of which specific meeting minutes will be reviewed, lest the IRB staff expend particular attention to those minutes. A program should conduct reviews at intervals sufficient to identify areas of concern and/or noncompliance as soon as possible. Doing so will help ensure that noncompliance is identified and resolved quickly. Such an approach also helps ensure that any reeducation, training, or coaching of IRB members or staff occurs in a timely manner. When resources are limited, a program may conduct such reviews only as needed or in direct response to reported or alleged noncompliance, an anticipated external inspection by FDA, a sponsor, or an accreditation site visit (e.g., AAHRPP).

- *Content*. An IRB file review will certainly include the IRB meeting minutes; however, it may also be helpful for the QA/QI reviewer to be familiar with the materials made available and distributed to IRB members for the IRB meeting. Although not a requirement, familiarity with the studies under review is likely to facilitate the review of the IRB meeting minutes. As such, a QA/QI reviewer may need access to the complete packet of materials provided to the IRB chair and/or primary IRB member in order to assess whether IRB members are receiving the appropriate materials and whether those materials are complete and provided in a timely manner.

- *Attendance at the IRB meeting*. Appointing a member of the QA/QI program to attend some or all IRB meetings is advantageous. Such a practice allows observation of the IRB "in action" and verification of subsequent documentation. Attendance also provides QA/QI staff with a better sense of the IRB's interpretation and application of regulations, which can prove useful when advising investigators. While the presence of QA/QI staff at an IRB meeting may further serve to facilitate the IRB review and approval process and ensure compliance, this type of involvement also has the potential to strain the relationship between the QA/QI program and the IRB. It can also divert resources from other necessary QA/QI activities, such as investigator site reviews. For these reasons, a program may wish to first assess whether potential noncompliance is likely to occur *during* the IRB meeting deliberations, or whether documentation is more likely to be at issue. If the latter, attendance at the IRB meeting may not provide significant benefit.

Table 5.3 depicts examples of common findings from an audit of IRB meeting minutes.

IRB Membership Composition Review

IRB membership is the backbone of the review and approval process. An IRB must be composed of members who have adequate training, education, and expertise. As a whole, the IRB should be sufficiently diverse and adequate in size to properly serve its research community. A QA/QI program is well-positioned to evaluate IRB member composition in order to ensure compliance with federal regulations (45 CFR 46.107 and 21 CFR 56.107) and applicable institutional policies and procedures. An example of an IRB Membership Composition Checklist can be found in the Appendix B.

Considerations for IRB Membership Composition Review

Although many of the considerations raised above relating to review of IRB files and meeting minutes apply to the review of IRB membership composition, the following points highlight some notable areas.

- *Periodicity*. To determine an appropriate schedule for reviewing IRB membership composition, a program should consider how often membership changes. Review of composition may be most valuable if implemented when membership changes occur or when an organization submits an IRB registration update/renewal to OHRP. Alternatively, a program may determine such a review will occur at regular intervals (e.g., on an annual basis). Such a strategy may be most appropriate for an organization with stable IRB membership.
- *Membership*. The IRB membership roster may appear in a variety of formats (e.g., Microsoft Word or Excel). A QA/QI program may also review available documentation collected by the IRB to demonstrate member qualifications, areas of expertise, and training (e.g., curriculum vitae, medical license, certificate(s) of completion for training received, and ethics training sessions attended or taught). Additionally, a QA/QI program may review membership to ensure there is appropriate expertise present on the committee (e.g., pediatrician on the IRB if research is routinely conducted with a pediatric population or prisoner representative if research involves prisons/prisoners).

Table 5.3. Examples of common findings from audit of IRB meeting minutes

Common findings	Applicable Regulations
IRB meeting minutes are not on file.	45 CFR 46.115(a)(2)* 21 CFR 56.115(a)(2)**
Attendance, including guests, recognized alternates, and/or consultants present not recorded or not accurately recorded.	45 CFR 46.115(a)(2)* 21 CFR 56.115(a)(2)**
Quorum and proper constitution for the meeting is not present or maintained for a convened meeting. Proper constitution for the meeting includes a scientist, non-scientist and non-affiliated member, or prisoner representative, if applicable.	45 CFR 46.108(b)* 21 CFR 56.107**
If permitted by institutional policy, meeting minutes do not record participation of IRB members by video or teleconference.	Minutes of Institutional Review Board (IRB)*** Meetings: Guidance for Institutions and IRBs (OHRP and FDA Joint Guidance; Sept. 2017)****
In relation to a motion, minutes do not record the number of members who voted for, against, or abstained.	45 CFR 46.115(a)(2)* 21 CFR 56.115(a)(2)**
Meeting minutes do not record IRB member recusal for potential conflict of interest, and when recused inaccurately includes them in the vote count.	45 CFR 46.107(e)* 21 CFR 56.107(e)**
Meeting minutes do not make clear that the required criteria for IRB approval have been satisfied.	45 CFR 46.111* 21 CFR 56.111**
Meeting minutes do not document that required elements of consent are present in ICF, or document alteration.	45 CFR 46.116* 45 CFR 46.117* 21 CFR 50 Subpart B**
Determinations not documented for waiver of consent or waiver of documentation of consent.	45 CFR 46.116(c)* 45 CFR 46.116(d)* 45 CFR 46.117(c)* 21 CFR 56.109(c)(1)** 21 CFR 56.109(c)(2)** 21 CFR 50.24**

This review should also include confirmation that the IRB roster maintained in the IRB office matches that on the IRB's registration with OHRP.

An Additional Note about Reviewer Neutrality

The reporting structure should not limit the ability of a QA/QI program to implement an IRB review function; however, as discussed in Chapter 2, forethought is necessary to determine how best to mitigate any

Common findings	Applicable Regulations
Determinations not documented related to IND or IDE determinations, including significant risk or nonsignificant risk determinations.	21 CFR 56.108(a)(1)** 21 CFR 812.66** 21 CFR 812.2(b)**
Meeting minutes do not document approval of use of short form consent process.	45 CFR 46.117(b)(2)* 21 CFR 50.27(b)(2)**
Meeting minutes do not document approval of enrollment of decisionally impaired persons, including approval of the assent/permission/consent process.	45 CFR 46.117(a)* 21 CFR 56.109(1)** 21 CRF 56.109(2)**
Failure to document IRB review of HHS grant application, as applicable. [Eliminated under new final rule, but still applies to those studies reviewed and approved under pre-2018 rule.]	45 CFR 46.120*
Meeting minutes insufficiently detail controverted issues discussed and their resolution.	45 CFR 46.115(a)(2)* 21 CFR 56.115(a)(2)**
A statement addressing frequency of IRB approval for new studies and those undergoing continuing review not present for each study.	45 CFR 46.109(e)* 45 CFR 56.109(f)*
Meeting minutes do not clearly identify whether changes required for approval are substantive or not and do not include sufficient detail to indicate the reason and the changes required.	45 CFR 46.115(a)(2)* 21 CFR 56.115(a)(2)** OHRP Guidance: Approval of Research with Conditions (Nov. 2010)
IRB Submissions (e.g., new studies, amendments, continuing review) processed via expedited review not reported to the convened IRB, including clarity related to frequency of IRB approval (e.g., for new studies, continuing review).	45 CFR 46.110(c)* 21 CFR 56.110(c)** 45 CFR 46.109(e)* 21 CFR 56.109(f)**
There is incomplete documentation of the determination and/or additional reporting requirements of unanticipated problems and/or serious or continuing noncompliance reviewed by the convened IRB.	45 CFR 46.115(a)(2)** 21 CFR 56.115(a)(2)* Minutes of Institutional Review Board (IRB) Meetings: Guidance for Institutions and IRBs (OHRP and FDA Joint Guidance; Sept. 2017)

*Office for Human Research Protections, "45 CFR 46 Protection of Human Subjects."
**U.S. Food and Drug Administration, "21 CFR 56 FDA Regulations Institutional Review Boards."
***Office for Human Research Protections, "Minutes of Institutional Review Board Meetings Guidance for Institutions and IRBs."
****Office for Human Research Protections, "Institutional Review Board Written Procedures: Guidance for Institutions and IRBs."

actual or perceived COI as well as to avoid any perception of COI within the research community.

Although QA/QI programs that are independent of IRB operations may be better positioned to objectively review IRB files, meeting minutes, or membership composition, there are ways to mitigate any perceived or actual COI regardless of a QA/QI program's structure. Programs can eliminate COI by having the IRB staff abstain from QA/QI review where s/he has also been responsible for IRB review-related duties. At smaller organizations, where separation of function may not be a feasible alternative, developing objective, standardized tools and checklists will help maintain consistency across reviews, diminish subjectivity, and facilitate a neutral review.

Post-review Follow-Up: Documenting Observations and Sharing Results

A QA/QI program should compile and document findings from its review of IRB files, meeting minutes, membership composition, and/or any other elements reviewed. This may take a variety of formats, ranging from a formal written report to an informal note-to-file. Consider the degree of formality of the report, as it may influence the interpretation of the review.

Regardless of the method implemented, the written record should sufficiently detail observations and, when appropriate, their suggested resolution. The latter may include both corrective actions and/or best practice recommendations or be summarized simply as general follow-up / next steps. When appropriate, consider providing an implementation deadline for each resolution, to ensure that findings are corrected in a timely manner. The QA/QI program should then track progress to ensure completion.

Sharing review findings with the IRB (including the IO, IRB chair(s), IRB director, and/or IRB staff) is critical to ensure compliance and facilitate improvement. Depending upon the office culture and the collaboration between the QA/QI program and the IRB, QA/QI and IRB program leadership should discuss effective methods of communicating findings, corrective actions, and/or best practice recommendations to IRB staff in order to achieve successful and timely resolutions. It is best if the initial dialogue about the plan for communication occurs in advance of the review, allowing for the plan to be modified thereafter. At the beginning of each review, the QA/QI staff should clarify who (e.g., IO, IRB chair) will receive the report and under what circumstances. For example, the findings of routine reviews might only be sent to the IRB chair and IRB director; however, any serious issue of noncompliance would also be sent to the IO.

It is helpful to determine, in advance if possible, who will be responsible for corrective action and follow-up, although additions or modifications to that plan may need to be made after a review is completed and findings identified. In some cases, organizational structure will largely dictate the appropriate person(s) to carry out these tasks. As an example, it may be natural for IRB staff to reconcile documentation when the IRB and QA/QI functions operate independently of one another. Under these circumstances, the QA/QI staff, however, may be better equipped to facilitate additional training and education and/or track outstanding items pending resolution. For smaller programs, where a single administrator many serve in a dual IRB-QA/QI capacity, it may be more efficient to correct the record in real time, i.e., during the IRB file review. As a result, although the written record would reflect the finding, the plan of action would likely denote "no further action," as the suggested corrective action would have been implemented. If changes to IRB meeting minutes are needed, an annotated document should be shared in advance of the next IRB meeting for deliberation and a vote at the meeting. Nevertheless, for transparency, all findings should be carefully documented in the IRB files.

Finally, a QA/QI program will need to address whether written records of IRB file reviews should become part of the IRB file and documentation or remain an internal QA/QI document. The nature of the findings may help determine where to retain the written record and report. For instance, a QA/QI program may elect to retain internal QA/QI documents unless potential serious or continuing noncompliance is observed, and, in the case of serious or continuing noncompliance, the written record would be sent to the IRB (and institutional leadership) and maintained within the IRB files or elsewhere.

SUMMARY

- QA/QI activities designed to evaluate IRB compliance include reviews of IRB files, meeting minutes, and membership composition.

- IRB file review can be complemented with an investigator site review for a comprehensive evaluation.

- When preparing to conduct an IRB file review, consider periodicity, access, scope, and content.

- A review of IRB membership composition should ensure the IRB is sufficiently diverse, adequate in size, and includes members with the necessary training, education, and expertise.

- A QA/QI program should compile and document findings from its review of IRB files, meeting minutes, and/or membership composition.

REFERENCES

1. US Food and Drug Administration, "21 CFR 56 FDA Regulations Institutional Review Boards"; Office for Human Research Protections, "45 CFR 46 Protection of Human Subjects"; Office of Human Research Protections, "Minutes of Institutional Review Board Meetings Guidance for Institutions and IRBs."

6

Metrics and Communicating Observations of Noncompliance

Leslie M. Howes and Sarah A. White

Purpose

In the course of QA/QI activities, a program collects a considerable amount of information. Protocol-specific observations are routinely shared with the investigator to facilitate corrective and/or preventive action(s) as necessary. IRB reviews will accumulate observations over time. In addition to looking at each investigator site review or IRB file review individually, aggregate data can be beneficial to the QA/QI program and to the larger institution. This chapter discusses protocol-specific and aggregate data collected by the QA/QI program, the potential utility of that data, and how best to communicate information to the research community.

Protocol-Specific Data

Protocol-specific data is typically provided to the investigator or study team to communicate details of a recent investigator site review. Feedback to investigators should identify any observations of noncompliance and provide specific examples, with an overall goal of self-directed, quality improvement.

Depending on institutional policies and procedures about the sharing of findings, all or some of the individual protocol data may be reported to the IRB. Individual reports to the IRB allow the IRB or IRB chair to assess noncompliance in relation to the approved protocol and request corrective action. The data, generally in the format of a report, should be provided within a short time frame after the onsite review (e.g., within two weeks). More detailed information regarding the format of an investigator site review report can be found in Chapter 4.

The QA/QI program should also consider, in consultation with institutional and IRB leadership, the threshold for when and how noncompliance identified during an investigator site review should be communicated and managed. These parameters must ensure that potential serious and/or continuing noncompliance is appropriately referred to the IRB. If there are other institutionally-defined events requiring an escalation plan, those should also be considered. While generally infrequent, serious or continuing noncompliance should be thoroughly investigated by the QA/QI program; specific details should be documented. An escalation plan, including the time frame for communicating such events to the IRB and/or institutional leadership should be defined. Depending on local policies and procedures, the QA/QI program may be assigned the task of working with the investigator to develop and implement corrective actions. Issues of confidentiality and records retention should be discussed with counsel prior to developing any written materials.

Aggregate Data

Aggregate data, or QA/QI metrics, combines all or some of the information gathered during study-specific, QA/QI activities and can be used to improve the overall compliance and quality of investigator and IRB performance and documentation.

It is important to collect QA/QI site review data in a consistent way to enable aggregate data analysis (Figure 6.1). A standardized observation index can assist in consistent data collection by categorizing findings across reviews. While details of unique observations may differ, the general observation (e.g., "study procedures were performed by individuals who lack IRB approval") should be the same (see Table 4.4). By reviewing these general, aggregated observations, QA/QI programs can identify common observations of investigator site or IRB file reviews. Common observations can then guide educational activities to increase awareness (e.g., presentations targeting either investigators or study staff).

Utilizing common observations can contribute to overall process improvement initiatives. This process starts with the QA/QI program determining the root cause of common observations. In doing so, the QA/QI program can better identify a solution that will correct and/or prevent future occurrence(s). Ideally, a QA/QI program will be able to continue to track

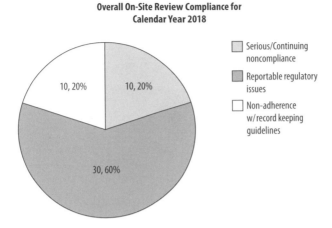

Overall On-Site Review Compliance for
Calendar Year 2018

10, 20%

10, 20%

30, 60%

- Serious/Continuing noncompliance
- Reportable regulatory issues
- Non-adherence w/record keeping guidelines

Figure 6.1. Example of investigator site review compliance metrics

any measures implemented to determine whether compliance has been achieved. See Figure 6.2 for an illustration of the process improvement.

As discussed in Chapter 4, the observations made during investigator site reviews may be of varying degrees of concern. Using a categorizing/grading system allows the program to quantify the seriousness of the observations. Grading systems can categorize each observation in terms of severity, frequency, and/or whether the observation would require reporting to the IRB. Alternatively, or in addition, a grading system can reflect the QA/QI investigator site review as a whole (i.e., may serve as a conclusion to the investigator site review, see Figure 4.2). When developing a categorizing/grading system, seek input and agreement from groups who will receive this information (e.g., IRB, research compliance, HRPP, and/or institutional leadership). The QA/QI program should also consider whether the grading system will be solely used for internal evaluation or will be reported to the research community or shared externally.

Once quantitative criteria have been assigned to observations and/or reviews, it is possible to generate comparative analyses and historical trending of the investigator site and IRB file reviews.

Observations and/or conclusions can be grouped by the following:

- Department
- Investigator

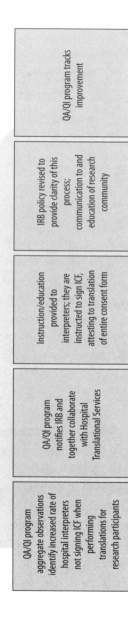

Figure 6.2. Example of steps to process improvement

QA/QI program aggregate observations identify increased rate of hospital interpreters not signing ICF when performing translations for research participants

QA/QI program notifies IRB and together collaborate with Hospital Translational Services

Instruction/education provided to interpreters; they are instructed to sign ICF, attesting to translation of entire consent form

IRB policy revised to provide clarity of this process; communication to and education of research community

QA/QI program tracks improvement

**Number of QA/QI Reviews and Education Sessions
FY 2016–2018**

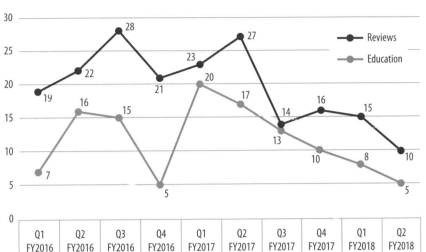

Figure 6.3. Example of QA/QI program service demand trends

- Sponsor
- Review type (e.g., convened IRB review or expedited)
- Site review type
- IRB panel/board
- IRB staff member or reviewer

QA/QI programs may also choose to track program service demand to understand trends in programmatic activity. This aids in development of new initiatives and anticipating resources. For example, Figure 6.3 shows a decrease in the number of education visits. This may reflect successful education in an area the QA/QI program has focused on for a given time period. Given the decrease in visits and expected increase in knowledge, the QA/QI program can adjust its efforts to address other areas of need. Further, such data can help inform personnel needs for the QA/QI program and may provide support for staffing additions/changes.

While aggregate information can be very useful to the research community in general (e.g., presentations of common findings), a QA/QI program should consider how broadly the information is or should be communicated. Posting common findings on a publicly-facing website or via

Table 6.1. Communicating QA/QI findings

Audience	Purpose of communicating findings	Metrics (examples)	Suggested format	Suggested timing
Investigators / study team	Communicate details of recent investigator site review Enable self-directed corrective / preventative action	General observation of noncompliance and specific examples	Written report	Immediately after the investigator site review (within 1–2 weeks)
Research community (investigators / staff)	Enable self-directed quality assurance / quality improvement	Frequent observations of noncompliance; best practices	Presentation	Annually
IRB chair or committee	Communicate details of recent audit Collaborate on corrective action plan	Common observations resulting from IRB file audits, IRB member composition evaluations, IRB minutes assessments, and IRB member qualification evaluations Common observations of investigator noncompliance Best practices	Written report	Immediately after the on-site review (within 1–2 weeks)
IRB leadership	Communicate noncompliance Identify gaps in institutional policies and procedures Collaborate on systemic improvement	Common observations resulting from IRB file audits, IRB member composition evaluations, IRB minutes assessments, and IRB member evaluations Common observations of investigator noncompliance Historical/comparative analysis of noncompliance over time	Presentation	Biannually

			Presentation	Biannually
Institutional (research) leadership	Provide pulse on noncompliance activity Inform about follow-up of major noncompliance Inform about systemic improvements Gain support for program activity	Specific observations about major non-compliance Aggregate metrics (historical/comparative analysis)	Presentation	Biannually
Accreditation organizations*	Provide metrics requested for accreditation standard	Audits of investigator protocols: # for-cause or directed # not-for-cause or random # site requested Audits of IRB records: # for-cause or directed # not-for-cause or random	Written report	Annually

*Association for the Accreditation of Human Research Protection Programs, Inc., "AAHRPP Annual Report."

an electronic newsletter may expose more information than the institution is comfortable sharing and/or may be misleading. Table 6.1 outlines suggested options for communicating QA/QI findings.

Identifying Best Practices

Though the majority of QA/QI findings are those of noncompliance, identifying "best practices" at research sites is another way of facilitating systemic improvements. Best practices can be policies or procedures put in place to ensure successful conduct and/or oversight of the study. They can and should be shared with both individual investigators and institutional leadership.

Communicating QA/QI Findings to Different Audiences

As described above, the data generated from investigator site and IRB file reviews can be utilized in a number of ways and communicated to different audiences at the institution. The QA/QI program should create a plan for how and when protocol-specific and aggregate data will be shared to ensure appropriate institutional stakeholders are informed of QA/QI activities and observations. Table 6.1 describes the various audiences as well as the purpose, format, and timing of communication. This plan can be incorporated into the institution's overall human research protection plan (HRPP) which will, in turn, give more value to the activities for which the QA/QI program is responsible.

SUMMARY

- Looking at aggregate data from investigator site reviews and IRB file reviews can be beneficial to the QA/QI program and institution at large.

- Feedback to investigators should identify any observations of noncompliance and provide specific examples, with an overall goal of self-directed, quality improvement.

- Common observations can be used to guide educational initiatives and changes to policies and procedures, thus creating an overall quality improvement process.

- QA/QI programs should develop a plan for communicating to the various stakeholders at their institution.

7

Educational Programming

Elizabeth Bowie and Leslie M. Howes

Purpose

Research practice and administration is governed by a constellation of international, federal, state, and local regulations. In addition, research and funding institutions require compliance with their own policies and procedures. Leveraging a QA/QI program to develop educational programming provides the necessary resources to facilitate compliance with relevant regulations and policies.

Educational outreach brings the QA/QI staff into the wider research community. The goal of such outreach should be to enhance the research process and foster open communication between research teams and the administration. Using the QA/QI program in this way may help dispel the perception of the QA/QI staff as the "compliance police." This chapter describes the educational function of a QA/QI program in terms of scope, audience, format, and content.

Scope

A QA/QI program may provide education to its entire research community, including researchers, study staff, research administrators, IRB members, and institutional officials. Alternatively, a QA/QI program may focus its outreach on certain key stakeholders (e.g., student investigators, IND-IDE holders). Education requirements are dictated by the research community's needs, institutional policy, and regulatory and funder requirements. QA/QI educational programs should reflect the needs of the institution. One size will not fit all: programs will vary depending on factors such as the type and breadth of the research portfolio, available resources, and institutional culture. Programs will also develop and change to reflect the dynamic needs of the audience.

Audiences

The key to a successful educational program is to know one's audience; the audience will dictate the content, tone, and complexity of a given program.

Educational programs can be designed for an audience of any composition or size. The audience size will influence the format choice, from an individual consultation to an institution-wide presentation. Some topics will draw a wide audience with varying backgrounds and knowledge. For example, the audience for a data safety presentation could be varied, including those who conduct social-behavioral-education research as well as those involved in biomedical research. If the background and educational attainment of the audience is varied, the content may need to be more general, and it may be more difficult to discuss the technical nuances of specific examples. A more targeted educational offering with an audience of similarly situated researchers (e.g., genetic researchers, researchers involved in IND/IDE studies) would allow for a far more specific and detailed presentation and interaction.

Formats

QA/QI educational programs can take many forms. Subject matter, audience size and composition, and institutional resources will help determine the best format (Table 7.1). Educational programs may be mandatory or voluntary. Mandatory programs are those that are required by institutional policy. The requirement(s) may be part of a scheduled training (e.g., new study staff orientation, annual compliance requirements) or the result of a newly identified problem (e.g., investigator noncompliance, required training in advance of sponsor-investigator IND/IDE approval).

In contrast, members of the research community may choose to engage in voluntary educational programs at their discretion. These types of programs may include a regularly scheduled series of talks that cover relevant topics (e.g., a quarterly lunchtime series covering topics of interest to research coordinators, such as "The Consent Process" or "Regulatory and/or

Table 7.1. Formats of QA/QI Educational Programming

Format	Utility	Audience/Considerations
Case study discussion	Exploring real-world problems to provide example issues of concern and possible solutions	Small- to medium-sized groups; attendees with similar expertise/baseline knowledge
Hands-on workshops/In-service training	Addressing a specific concern; program staff might provide tips and examples of how to develop SOPs or customized self-audit tools	Small- to medium-sized groups; attendees with similar expertise/baseline knowledge
Office hours	Addressing the research community's questions in a relaxed atmosphere; gaining insight into the community's regulatory challenges; offering the community opportunities to meet program staff	1-on-1 and small-sized groups; both experienced and novice researchers should be encouraged to attend
Educational series	Discussing relevant QA/QI topics, either in person or via regularly scheduled newsletters	Small- to medium-sized groups; having attendees who share a common research background is helpful to ensure the series addresses the target audience's educational needs
"Mock" site visit	Showing researchers/staff what to expect from and how to prepare for a site visit/external audit	Small-sized group with similar expertise/baseline knowledge
Virtual trainings	Engaging with a wide range of researchers over a dispersed geographic area	Large groups with diverse research backgrounds; useful for multicenter studies; international research teams
Website	Providing a home for QA/QI tools and resources and ensuring resources are readily available to the research community	Broad audience
Newsletters	Announcing upcoming events or educational series; highlighting regulations impacting researchers and staff	Broad audience
Educational opportunities during the QA/QI process	Augmenting or supplementing site reviews, IRB file reviews, setup programs, etc., with just-in-time information presented formally or informally	1-on-1

Policy Updates"). Additionally, sending out scheduled newsletters can be an easy method of disseminating information to researchers about new regulations or upcoming educational offerings (Figure 7.1).

Common Topics Covered

As described above, whenever possible, the content of educational programming should be tailored to the audience, focused, and limited to what the audience needs to know. For example, if the audience consists of researchers who conduct social-behavioral-education research, then a discussion of the Common Rule would be appropriate. However, there would be no need to provide an in-depth explanation of FDA regulations; a passing reference to the fact that FDA regulations and the Common Rule mirror one another (perhaps with a citation) is likely sufficient. Focusing programming in this way demonstrates a mutual respect for the limited time and resources of researchers, administrators, and QA/QI professionals.

A variety of resources can help QA/QI programs identify appropriate topics for educational programming:

- *QA/QI On-Site Reviews*. QA/QI on-site reviews provide a wealth of information regarding the educational needs of the research community. When reviewing the findings from on-site reviews, QA/QI program staff should look for patterns that indicate further education is required (see Chapter 6). Once a gap is identified, the program may then determine the best format in which to offer education to address that gap (e.g., as an in-service training to the department or as a talk that is open to a wider audience).
- *IRB Administration*. The QA/QI staff might consider speaking to the IRB to determine if they have identified trends in protocol submissions that indicate further education is needed. For example, when introducing a new policy on data security, IRB reviewers may observe that submitted IRB applications/protocols are frequently incomplete or insufficient in outlining appropriate provisions to comply with the policy.
- *IRB Reportable Events Submissions*. A review of the reportable events submitted to the IRB might reveal a pattern of protocol deviations or noncompliance that could be prevented by implementing proactive education.

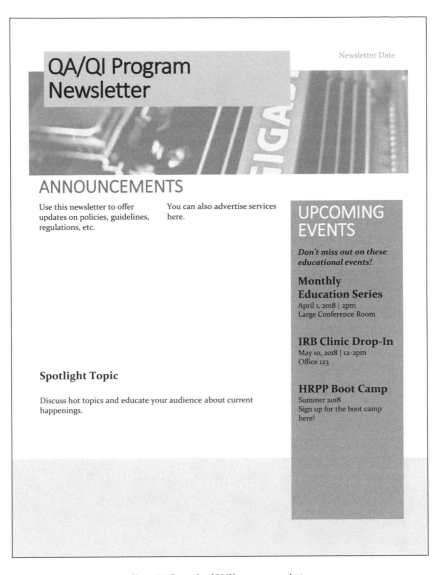

Figure 7.1. Example of QA/QI program newsletter

- *Researchers*. Researchers might identify topics on which they would like more information. For example, a researcher deciding to expand his or her recruitment to include participants from a new ethnic group may request a presentation regarding consent of non-English speaking subjects. Such a presentation may include information regarding translating forms, using the short form consent, and exercising cultural competency.

- *Institutional Leadership.* QA/QI programs should consult with institutional leadership (e.g., IRB chairs, IO) to determine if there are perceived gaps in investigator or staff knowledge; this assessment could be done as part of the annual evaluation of the IRB, IRB members, or chairs.
- *Regulatory Updates.* Whenever there are changes to regulations, the QA/QI program should develop, in collaboration with the IRB Office, educational outreach programs to ensure that everyone in the research community who may need to know about the changes has access to information about the regulatory changes, and understands the implications of those changes.

Common Presentation Topics

- Is my research exempt?
- How the federal regulations protect research participants
- The human subjects research approval process: from initial application to termination
- How to draft consent text for an online survey
- HIPAA, PHI, and research
- Regulatory documentation requirements for FDA-regulated and non-FDA-regulated research
- Obtaining and documenting informed consent
- Obtaining and documenting assent from minors and permission from parents/guardians
- Identifying and assessing adverse events
- Audits and inspections from external sponsors
- Sponsor-investigator documentation
- Database of Genotypes and Phenotypes (dbGAP) submissions and institutional certification
- Institution-specific trainings on policies, procedures, and the IRB process
- How to avoid common noncompliance
- IRB submission requirements
- Regulation changes
- Impact of new legislation on human subjects research

Planning and Execution

QA/QI staff must identify the different types of research being conducted at the institution so that they can identify the governing regulatory requirements. Next, the program designers need to incorporate the institution's policies. The program must be designed with a clear view of the expectations of senior management regarding research education. Incorporating institutional expectations early in the design of an educational program establishes a solid foundation and increases efficiency.

For many QA/QI programs, resources are scarce. QA/QI programs must work efficiently, but creatively, with the available tools and resources to develop the most responsive educational offerings. It is important to develop collaborative relationships within the research community and the institution, and to leverage strengths, resources, and knowledge whenever appropriate.

The benefit of working with collaborators is twofold. First, the presence of collaborators indicates support from the community. Whenever institutional officials and staff are involved in a QA/QI program's educational offerings, the message is clear that the QA/QI program and educational offering has the support of the institution. Likewise, the collaboration of investigators and staff in a QA/QI educational program demonstrates that the investigators see value in the QA/QI program. Second, collaborators can provide practical "on-the-ground" feedback that the program can incorporate into richer, and more effective, offerings. Collaborators can provide information that will help in planning future educational programs and targeting research communities.

Collaborators may include

- *Researchers / Study Staff.* Working directly with the research community will help QA/QI program staff better address the community's specific needs. A program may solicit study staff to collaborate on educational offerings; such collaborations can range in size and form and may be program-initiated or researcher-initiated. The researcher / study staff may work side-by-side in a very hands-on way to develop the educational offering, or the researcher may simply provide the topic and ask the program to develop the presentation. As a result of the collaboration, the QA/QI staff will likely better understand the research topic and have forged valuable connections with the individuals in the group.

EXAMPLE: The IRB has identified a research coordinator who has a talent for crafting simple and concise consent forms. The QA/QI program staff might contact her and ask if she would help in a presentation on drafting consent forms. That coordinator could present as a guest speaker in a series of scheduled talks or simply attend a talk to field questions, offer tips, and provide a working perspective, while the QA/QI program staff speak to regulatory/institutional requirements. In addition, the coordinator might help draft the presentation for the educational series or help develop a standalone presentation to be available on the QA/QI program website.

- *Institutional/Departmental Collaboration.* Both academic and administrative departments should be considered as possible collaborators. Academic department leadership may be able to identify an educational need based on past experiences or future research plans. They may also be in the best position to address a policy that is particularly relevant to their research agenda. Administrative collaborators include the offices of human resources (HR), sponsored programs, and research integrity, a conflict of interest committee, or quality and safety departments.

EXAMPLE 1: In certain cases, the QA/QI program might ask HR to provide the contact information of new employees who will be working in research (often identified by job title), in order to engage this subset of employees individually or as a group to ensure that the new employees are aware of the QA/QI program offerings and to provide more research-specific programming. By collaborating with HR, the program may reach a wide and relevant audience in a timely and methodical manner.

EXAMPLE 2: Sponsored programs (grants and contracts) administrators may be another appropriate group from which to select institutional partners and administrative collaborators. Often, funding proposals are submitted early in the process of study initiation and grants or funding contacts have a responsibility to know which federal regulations and institutional policies are relevant to their review. Providing education about IRB review, exemptions, and other information can help this group identify studies that may need IRB review as well as help to catch issues prior to study initiation.

Even the most spectacular educational initiative fails if the intended audience cannot or does not access the information. Once the educational program is designed, it must be effectively and appropriately advertised, including the use of e-mails, fliers, newsletters, and even tent cards on lunch tables. Any website or blog maintained by the QA/QI program or the IRB office should include a section for advertising the educational offerings.

What Next? Evaluation and Improvement

Education is an ongoing process. After each educational offering, a QA/QI program should take the opportunity to evaluate the offering and use the data to change programming as needed. Participant evaluations can be gathered through online or paper-based surveys. In order to evaluate the effectiveness of a QA/QI program's educational offerings, try to collect metrics on immediate and future outcomes, including the following:

- Attendee demographics
- Evaluation of session topic/speakers/logistics (e.g., time of day, duration, etc.)
- Whether investigators who attend educational programs obtain IRB approval more quickly
- Whether investigators who attend educational programs submit fewer reportable events to the IRB
- Whether labs or groups whose members attend educational programs perform better at site visits

Programs should share these metrics with the research community and use the data to evaluate past programming and design future offerings. The educational function of a QA/QI program is not static. It should evolve and change based on the needs of the institution and its researchers.

SUMMARY

- The goal of a QA/QI program's educational outreach is to enhance the research process and foster open communication between research teams and the HRPP.

- The content of educational programming should be tailored to the audience and limited to what the target audience needs to know.

- A QA/QI program should evaluate its educational offerings and use the data to change programming as needed.

Appendix A
Abbreviations and Acronyms

AAHRPP	Association for the Accreditation of Human Research Protection Programs
AE	adverse event
CAPA	corrective and preventive actions
COI	conflicts of interest
CV	curriculum vitae
DbGaP	Database of Genotypes and Phenotypes
DMC	Data Monitoring Committee
FDA	US Food and Drug Administration
FTE	full-time employee
GAO	General Accounting Office
GCP	good clinical practice
HHS	US Department of Health and Human Services
HIPAA	Health Insurance Portability and Accountability Act
HRPP	Human Research Protection Program
IAA	IRB authorization agreement
ICH	International Council for Harmonisation
IDE	investigational device exemption
IND	investigational new drug
IO	institutional official
IRB	Institutional Review Board
NIH	National Institutes of Health
NTF	note-to-file
OCR	Office of Civil Rights, HHS
OHRP	Office for Human Research Protections, HHS
OIG	Office of the Inspector General
P&P	policies and procedures
PHI	protected health information
PI	principal investigator
QA/QI	quality assurance / quality improvement

QIP	quality improvement program
SAE	serious adverse event
SBER	social-behavioral-education research
SR	significant risk (in IDE regulations)

Appendix B
Resources

Chapter 2

Job Description: QA/QI Specialist

SCOPE OF POSITION

Under the direction of the Managing Director, the incumbent is responsible for providing high-level human research support service to the research community, including faculty members and students. The incumbent is required to work independently with minimal supervision and is responsible for determining when to refer situations/issues to leadership.

PRINCIPLE DUTIES

- Provide front-line support and information for customers of the quality improvement program (QIP), including faculty, students, and staff regarding its services and tools.
- Develop and deliver educational curriculum for the research community by request and when initiated by the IRB and/or QIP (both domestically and abroad).
- Conduct on-site reviews (both domestically and abroad) to ensure regulatory compliance including protocol adherence, accurate record keeping, and appropriate informed consent processing of human subjects research.
- Draft, edit, and prepare correspondence, reports, study management tools, and other material using word processing, spreadsheets, and/or databases.
- Contribute to office goals by accomplishing other related duties as required and assigned by the institution, e.g., accreditation activities, participant outreach activities, etc.

QUALIFICATIONS

- Bachelor's degree required; Master's degree in related field preferred.
- Minimum of three years experience in research administration, quality improvement, or another related field.

- Must obtain the Certified IRB Professional (CIP) designation or be CIP eligible. If the successful applicant does not already possess the CIP designation, he/she will be required to obtain it within one year of start date.
- Solid understanding of federal and state regulations governing human research.
- Strong analytical, written, and oral communication skills and ability to multitask in a busy office environment while maintaining superior customer service.
- Ability to use multiple technical applications including word processing, database management, spreadsheets, graphics and presentation software, electronic calendar, e-mail, and other technical applications.
- Ability to maintain strict standards of confidentiality.
- Excellent verbal and written communication skills.

Chapter 3
Policy Manual Template
SAMPLE QA/QI POLICY MANUAL

Below is a sample QA/QI policy manual template that may be useful as a starting point when drafting your own policies and procedures. Policy manuals generally follow a generic format that begins with an introduction, including mission, aims, and goals; program scope; an overview; and definitions. These sections are then broken down by topic and include a policy statement and procedures that support the given policy. When writing the QA/QI policy manual, some additional drafting points to consider include the following:

- Be concise; state your policies clearly and avoid unnecessary words and concepts.
- Demystify the process and make your activities transparent to the community; provide step-by-step instructions so that the intended audience can understand what will happen and what their roles and responsibilities will be.
- Periodically review and revise policies to reflect changes in practice; many organizations implement an annual review to capture changes in law, practice, and personnel.

This sample QA/QI policy manual was created by reviewing the QA/QI policies and/or procedures from a number of institutions: Boston Children's Hospital, Cambridge Health Alliance, Harvard T. H. Chan School of Public Health, the University of Pittsburgh, the University of California San Francisco, and the University of Michigan.

Depending on your organizational culture and program structure, you may find that not all of the policies delineated below apply and/or other policies may be required. The following sample is intended as a guide and should be augmented to meet the needs of your program and institution.

SAMPLE TABLE OF CONTENTS FOR QA/QI PROGRAM POLICY
1. **Policy**
   [Concise statement describing what will be accomplished]
2. **Purpose and background for policy**
   a. [Brief statement of the intention of the policy]
   b. Why is the policy in place?

      i. Regulations

      ii. Benefits

      iii. How it helps achieve institutional or program aims and goals

      iv. Describe any problems or conflicts the policy hopes to address

3. **Application**
   a. To whom does this policy apply?
   b. Who is the audience?

4. **Responsible parties**
   a. Who has authority to enforce the policy?
   b. Who reviewed and approved the policy?
   c. What is the date of approval?
   d. When will the policy be re-reviewed?

5. **Introduction**
   a. Mission, aims, and goals
   b. Program scope and responsibilities
       [Insert description of institutional support and specific program responsibilities]
   c. General overview of services
       [List of program services and activities with very brief summary and/or reference to more detailed policy]
   d. Definitions
       [List common terms, abbreviations, and definitions that may not be obvious or are specific to institution]

6. **Investigator/study reviews**
   a. Routine/not-for-cause site reviews
       i.   Process for identifying studies and random selection instructions
       ii. Investigator self-assessments/checklists
       iii. Review of file in advance of compliance activity
   b. Directed/for-cause site review
   c. Review process: PI and research staff

7. **Review and management of post-approval event reports**
   a. HRPP post approval reporting requirements
   b. Procedures for assessment and review and IRB determination
   c. Reporting

8. **Investigation of allegations and findings of noncompliance**

a. Purpose, scope, and responsibilities

b. Procedures

c. Investigation

d. Notification to investigators of allegations

e. Review, determination, documentation, and management of serious and/or continuing noncompliance

f. Appeals process

9. **HRPP reporting requirements for unanticipated problems, serious and/or continuing noncompliance, suspension, or termination of approved research**

a. Purpose, scope, and responsibilities

b. Preparation and distribution of letter to the PI

c. Preparation and distribution of the report

d. Time frame for reporting

e. Follow-up reports

10. **Feedback: Evaluation of the HRPP and IRB**

a. QA/QI program review

b. Program awareness

c. Incorporating the findings of routine site reviews, directed or for-cause site reviews, and internal QI reviews

d. Reviewing and analyzing HRPP participant survey responses

e. Analyzing and recommending improvements for the coordination and efficiencies of the different offices, committees, and individuals responsible for HRPP at the institution

11. **Other topics**

a. Sponsor-investigator pre-review (IND/IDE)

   i. IND sponsor-investigator responsibilities

   ii. IDE significant risk (SR) device sponsor-investigator responsibilities

   iii. IDE non-significant risk (NSR) device sponsor-investigator responsibilities

b. Subject outreach

c. New investigator review/pre-review

   i. New/transfer PI meeting checklist

   ii. New/transfer PI meeting handouts and guidance

12. **References**

[List any references (e.g. regulations, other policies) or related content that may help the audience better understand policy or provide background. If possible, add hyperlinks to facilitate easy referencing.]

13. **Definitions**

[Define any unique and/or technical terms that will help the audience understand the policy]

14. **Document attributes**

Author

Date of approval and subsequent review dates

Revisions described, if applicable

Example

Author/Owner	*[e.g., Department Chair]*	
Approved by		
Approval Date	*[1/1/20XX]*	
Effective Date	*[1/1/20XX]*	
Review Date(s):	*[1/1/20XX]*	☐ Revisions made, *specify:*
	[1/1/20XX]	☐ Revisions made, *specify:*
	[1/1/20XX]	☐ Revisions made, *specify:*

Sample SOP: Directed Audit (For-Cause Audit)

1 Purpose

1.1 This procedure establishes the process for QIP to conduct directed audits.

1.2 The process begins when the IRB/Institutional Official (I/O) has identified the need for directed audit. Directed audits may be conducted in response to participant or sponsor complaints, requests from Harvard Chan School or HMS institutional officials, IRB Chairs, or concerns from government agencies (e.g., FDA, NIH, and OHRP).

1.3 The process ends when QIP has provided a formal report and recommended corrective actions / quality improvement suggestions to the investigator and IRB/IO.

2 Revisions from Previous Version

2.1 None.

3 Policy

3.1 QIP conducts domestic and international directed audits of study documentation to ensure regulatory compliance including protocol adherence, accurate record keeping, and appropriate informed consent process.

3.2 QIP provides corrective actions and offers quality improvement suggestions to facilitate best practices and enhance overall study conduct.

4 Responsibilities

4.1 QIP Staff are responsible for carrying out these procedures.

5 Procedure

5.1 Schedule a directed audit with the investigator and additional members of the study staff when appropriate.

If the Harvard LMA School has been designated as the IRB of Record under the Harvard Catalyst Common Reciprocal Reliance Agreement, notify the Director or designee (see Catalyst Designated Contacts list) prior to conducting the audit via email providing: PI name, Protocol number, Protocol Title, date of audit, and reason for audit.

5.2 Review corresponding IRB file and prepare onsite review tools using the "CHECKLIST: Audit Tool" as a guide.

5.3   Review electronic and hard copy regulatory documentation and participant files (sample when appropriate) available onsite or remotely.

5.4   When possible, conduct an exit interview with the Principal Investigator (PI) and/or designee. Provide investigator and additional members of the study staff with preliminary findings and an opportunity to correct, explain, and/or ask questions.

5.5   Communicate audit findings to the investigator and IRB, and/or Harvard LMA School institutional officials, as appropriate, within 5 business days using "TEMPLATE LETTER: Directed Audit Letter" and, when appropriate, "TEMPLATE LETTER: Directed Audit Report."

5.6   Discuss findings and recommendations with IRB Assistant Director, OHRA Managing Director, and/or IO, as appropriate.

5.7   If Harvard LMA School has been designated as the IRB of Record under the Harvard Catalyst Common Reciprocal Reliance Agreement, notify the Director or designee (see Catalyst Designated Contacts list) of audit completion within 30 days using the Catalyst Audit Notification/Closure form.

5.8   Conduct IRB File Audit as appropriate, "CHECKLIST: IRB File Observations–Resolution Chart"

5.9   Follow the "SOP: QIP Records" and "SOP: IRB Records" to file correspondence.

5.10 Work with investigator to implement best practice recommendations and required corrective actions.

5.11 If appropriate, send a copy to any government agencies (e.g., FDA, NIH, and OHRP), if required.

6 Materials

6.1   CHECKLIST: Audit Tool

6.2   TEMPLATE LETTER: Directed Audit Letter

6.3   TEMPLATE LETTER: Directed Audit Report

6.4   CHECKLIST: IRB File Observations–Resolution Chart

6.5   SOP: QIP Records

6.6   SOP: IRB Records

7 References

7.1   None.

Sample SOP: Routine On-Site Review (Not-for-Cause Audit)

1 Purpose

1.1 This procedure establishes the process for QIP to conduct routine on-site review.

1.2 The process begins when the investigator and/or study staff has requested routine on-site review or the protocol has been identified as per OHRA's criteria for QIP-initiated routine on-site review (e.g., new/transfer PIs).

1.3 The process ends when QIP has communicated the review findings in writing to the investigator.

2 Revisions from Previous Version

2.1 None.

3 Policy

3.1 OHRA staff conduct domestic and international routine on-site review of study documentation to ensure regulatory compliance including protocol adherence, accurate record keeping, and appropriate informed consent process.

3.2 QIP provides corrective actions and offers quality improvement recommendations to facilitate best practices and enhance overall study conduct.

4 Responsibilities

4.1 QIP Staff are responsible for carrying out these procedures.

5 Procedure

5.1 Schedule routine on-site review with the investigator and/or additional members of the study staff when appropriate.

5.2 If Harvard LMA School has been designated as the IRB of Record under the Harvard Catalyst Common Reciprocal Reliance Agreement, notify the Director or designee (see Catalyst Designated Contacts list) prior to conducting the review via e-mail providing: PI name, Protocol Number, Protocol Title, date of audit, reason for audit.

5.2 Complete an IRB file review in preparation of going on-site.

5.3 Review electronic and hard copy regulatory documentation and (sample) participant files available on-site or remotely.

5.4 When possible, conduct an exit interview with the Principal Investigator and/or designee. Provide investigator and additional members of the study staff with preliminary findings and an opportunity to correct, explain, and/or ask questions.

5.5   Communicate review findings with the investigator within 5 business days via e-mail and, when appropriate, "TEMPLATE LETTER: On-site Review Report."

5.6   If Harvard LMA School has been designated as the IRB of Record under the Harvard Catalyst Common Reciprocal Reliance Agreement, notify the Director or designee (see Catalyst Designated Contacts list) of review completion within 60 days using the Catalyst Audit Notification/Closure form.

5.7   Conduct IRB File Audit as appropriate, "CHECKLIST: IRB File Observations-Resolution Chart"

5.8   Follow the "SOP: QIP Records" to file correspondence to and from QIP.

5.9   Work with the investigator to implement best practice recommendations and required corrective actions, when appropriate.

6 Materials

6.1   TEMPLATE LETTER: On-site Review Report

6.2   CHECKLIST: IRB File Observations-Resolution Chart

6.3   SOP: QIP Records

7 References

7.1   None.

Chapter 4
Audit Certificate Template

[Organization Logo]

Date: [Date of issuing audit certificate]

Audit Certificate

Protocol #:

[Protocol Number]

Protocol Title:

[Protocol Title]

THIS CERTIFIES THAT

[Name/Title of PI]

[Work Address of PI]

HAS UNDERGONE A DETAILED AUDIT [Contents of the audit. Subjects and summarization of findings, trial, chemical name, identification code, identification drug, etc.]

Auditor

[Name and title of auditor]

[signature of auditor]

[Work address of auditor]

[City, state, zip]

Auditor Manager

[Name and title of auditor manager]

[signature of auditor]

[Work address of auditor]

[City, state, zip]

Investigator Site Review Report Template

Protocol Title:	*[Protocol Title]*
Principal Investigator:	*[Name]*
	[Department, School]
Funding Source:	*[Funding Source]*
Date of Review:	*[Date]*
Auditors:	*[Name(s)]*
Date of Report:	*[Date]*
Distribution:	*[PI Name]*

I. INTRODUCTION:

[include brief introduction, suggested details to include: purpose of site review, who was present, etc.]

II. STUDY SUMMARY:

[Include brief summary of the study being audited.]

III. SCOPE OF REVIEW:

[Include all material reviewed including regulatory documentation, consent forms, subject files, etc.]

The following documents were reviewed during the audit:

IV. REGULATORY REVIEW HISTORY:

OVERALL FINDINGS:
[Include summary of observations in bulleted format with sufficient detail and outline any specific findings below.]

SPECIFIC QIP FINDINGS:

Observations	Corrective Actions / Best Practice Recommendations
Regulatory Documentation	Corrective Action:
	Best Practice Recommendation:
Informed Consent	Corrective Action:
	Best Practice Recommendation:
Participant Files	Corrective Action:
	Best Practice Recommendation:

V. CONCLUSIONS:
[Summarize the site review and provide contact for questions; if response from site is required, identify timeline for response.]

Short Audit Spot Check Template

[logo]   **SHORT AUDIT FORM FOR IRB APPROVED PROJECTS**

	IRB Number	Site of Audit	Date of Audit
Review Category:	☐ Exempt _____	☐ Expedited _____	☐ Full Board Review
Title of Project:			

This audit is based on information submitted on the renewal application dated *[insert MM/DD/YYYY]*.
Number of subjects recruited since the last approval period: _____

Research Study Team (Key personnel)		
Name	**Role**	**Is training current?**
	Principal Investigator	☐ Yes ☐ No
		☐ Yes ☐ No
		☐ Yes ☐ No
		☐ Yes ☐ No
		☐ Yes ☐ No
		☐ Yes ☐ No
		☐ Yes ☐ No
		☐ Yes ☐ No
		☐ Yes ☐ No

Consent Forms	
All consent forms are correctly filed and accounted for.	☐ Yes ☐ No If no, explain:
All consent forms are signed and dated accurately.	☐ Yes ☐ No If no, explain:
All consent forms used are from an approved version.	☐ Yes ☐ No If no, explain:
Comments:	

Data collection	
All data collection instruments were approved versions.	☐ Yes ☐ No If no, explain:
All physical and/or electronic data is kept in secure location according to application.	☐ Yes ☐ No If no, explain:
Comments:	

Additional Comments		
Auditor(s) name and signature(s)	Time started: _____	Time ended: _____

[Insert name and signature/date of auditor(s).]

PI Notification Letter Template

To: *[Principal Investigator]*
From: *[Requester]*
Date: *[Date]*
Re: **Quality Improvement Review Notification for Protocol**
         [PROTOCOL #: PROTOCOL TITLE]

In accordance with [institution name] policy, the [QA/QI program name] conducts on-time study reviews of randomly selected, active protocols involving human subjects. One goal of the study review is to help investigators / research staff implement tools and strategies to improve upon identified problem areas. When possible, *[QA/QI program name]* will provide educational materials, support, and tools.

You are being contacted at this time because **Protocol** *[protocol #]* has been selected for review.

While this review is required, please note that the findings and observations will be *kept confidential* between the PI and the QA/QI office. Only in the event that a serious deviation is discovered will the IRB be notified as to determine a plan of action to best resolve the issue.

To help you prepare for the audit, it is strongly suggested that you conduct a self-assessment of the study. You may refer to the Investigator Self-Assessment Checklist to help you with that process.

Please reference the Quality Improvement Review Summary document, as it provides a list of the study documents that should be available for review and a general outline of the review process.

We will contact you within the next week to set up an initial meeting and monitoring visit with the hope to complete the review within 1 month. After the monitoring visit, a final meeting will be scheduled to discuss preliminary findings and to answer any questions or concerns. A final report will be sent to you within 2 weeks of the final meeting. All pertinent research staff (e.g., co-investigators, research coordinators / nurses) involved in this protocol are encouraged to participate in the Initial and Exit Meetings.

The QA/QI program is dedicated to providing education and support to researchers involved in the conduct of safe, compliant, and high-quality human research. Your participation is appreciated, and we look forward to working with you and your research team.

If you have any questions or concerns, or if you would like to go ahead and schedule the review, please contact [contact name] at [insert e-mail and/or telephone number].

Regards,
[name of Auditor]
[include CC'ed personnel]

PI Response Form Template

CONFIDENTIAL
Study Review: Principal Investigator Response Form

Instructions: The contents of this form are **CONFIDENTIAL**. The PI must review, address, and respond to each **Required Action** and **Recommend Action** as outlined. Do not include any PHI in this report. Please return this form to the auditor according to the due date below. If you have any questions, please contact *[insert contact information]*.

Part A. Required Actions: *all actions must be addressed promptly* to meet federal regulations, guidelines and *[insert institution]* policies. If the required action is not possible or cannot be completed, please provide reason.

Part B. Recommended Actions: consider all recommended actions. While not mandatory, it is strongly encouraged to consider the recommendations, evaluate them in terms of your program/study procedures and to incorporate as deemed helpful.

Please respond to each recommendation with one of the following actions:

→ Accept Action	Recommendation deemed useful and action implemented. Please explain how.
→ Postpone Action	Recommendation deemed useful, but action will be implemented later in this study and/or will be applied to future studies.
→ Decline Action	Recommendation deemed impractical or unfeasible for this study as well as future studies.
→ Acknowledge	As applicable, an observation may be noted in which no follow-up action is necessary, but PI will be asked to acknowledge or clarify.

Once this form is complete, please sign below and return (PDF by e-mail) to [insert e-mail] by the due date.

STUDY INFORMATION

Principal Investigator:

Protocol Number:

Protocol Title:

PI RESPONSE DUE DATE:

Part A. REQUIRED ACTIONS: all actions must be addressed promptly

Ref.	Required Action	PI Response	EXPLAIN RESPONSE (COMPLETED: If no changes, no response required; OTHER / NO ACTION: Why alternative or no action taken; ACKNOWLEDGED: As applicable, acknowledge or clarify)
A1		☐ COMPLETED ☐ OTHER / NO ACTION	Response:
A2		☐ COMPLETED ☐ OTHER / NO ACTION	Response:
A3		☐ COMPLETED ☐ OTHER / NO ACTION	Response:

Part B. RECOMMENDED ACTIONS: consider all recommendations

Ref.	Recommended Action	PI Response	EXPLAIN RESPONSE (ACCEPT: Describe action taken and when; POSTPONE: Why action will be implemented in future; DECLINE: Why action not taken; ACKNOWLEDGE: As applicable, acknowledge or clarify)
B1		☐ ACCEPT ☐ POSTPONE ☐ DECLINE	Response:
B1		☐ ACCEPT ☐ POSTPONE ☐ DECLINE	Response:
B1		☐ ACCEPT ☐ POSTPONE ☐ DECLINE	Response:

COMMENTS

This signature indicates the Principal Investigator has reviewed this report, shared findings and provided copies to appropriate research staff and addressed all Required and Recommended Actions.

Principal Investigator (Printed): _____

Principal Investigator Signature: _____   **Date:** _____

PI Site Review Summary Template

QUALITY IMPROVEMENT REVIEW SUMMARY

The following information outlines what to expect during a routine (not-for-cause) audit. This is a general description and is subject to change based on factors such as type of research and availability. While this audit is required, we will work with you throughout the process to ensure the process goes smoothly and when needed, can be flexible to accommodate schedules.

If you have any questions, please contact *[insert contact information]*.

Pre-Meeting Responsibilities

1. Provide a list of all enrolled participants (without names or other PHI). The auditor will select specific subject files for audit. The list of selected files will be provided to you in advanced so please have their complete study file/binder available for review. At the time of audit, additional records maybe requested for review.

2. Please have all study and participant documents, binders, and files available at the time of review. If any of these documents are stored electronically (e.g., SharePoint, REDCap, department shared drive), please do not make paper copies for the purposes of this review. We will send a checklist before the audit asking where documents are stored and if electronic, how we will be able to access at the time of the audit.

This may include any of the following:

- IRB Documentation (e.g., submissions, action letters, PI responses, approval letters, acknowledgments, unanticipated event reports, significant deviations)
- Signed consent forms (current and expired versions)
- Management and/or monitoring logs
- Participant recruitment material
- Research team staff training
- Study records (including participant eligibility determination & documentation and screening procedures)

- Study procedures (including conduct & documentation of procedures)
- On-site record keeping (including storage of documents and participant files)
- Regulatory documentation for Investigational Drug/Device trials (if applicable)

3. Ensure there will be available space (e.g. desk or room) for the auditor at the time of the review. The auditor will need space to review the study documents on the date schedule. Depending on the study and the number of participants, the review can last a few hours or need to be conducted over a few days.

SUMMARY OF REVIEW PROCESS

Initial Meeting with Principal Investigator ~30–45 minutes

1. **The auditor will present a summary and explain the review process.**
   The PI and staff will be encouraged to ask questions throughout.
2. **The auditor will ask study specific questions.**
   The questions will pertain to study information not easily observed from study documents and regarding actual study practices.
3. **The PI and staff will be encouraged to ask questions and provide feedback.**
   The PI and research staff will be given the opportunity to ask any questions and offer opinions about the review and other question about the QA/QI program.
4. **Final Meeting Scheduled**
   Ideally scheduled at the end of the Study/Subject Review or within 1 week of meeting, at which time any study findings will be reviewed with PI and staff.

Study and Subject Records Review ~4–6 hours (depending on study)

1. **The auditor will review provided study and subject materials in the reserved space.**
   PI and staff do not need to be present, but please have one study

staff available via phone/page. Once the review is complete, study files/records will be returned as instructed by research team.

Note: The length of the Routine Audit is dependent on many factors such as the type of study, how long the study has been open, number of subjects enrolled. We do aim to complete the review of study and subject files within 1 day. To facilitate this, we try to schedule the start time during the morning. If we think the review may take longer, we will let you know as soon as possible.

Final Meeting ~45 minutes–1 hour

1. **QI Specialist will review the findings and observations noted from the review.**
   At this time, the research staff can make any clarifications as needed. If there are findings and/or observations, they will be broken into three categories:

   ■ **Notable Best Practices**: Study strengths will be highlighted.
   ■ **Require Corrective Actions**: Corrective actions required to meet regulations and policies.
   ■ **Recommended Actions**: Actions to be considered if PI feels them beneficial to the study.

2. **PI and Research Staff will be encouraged to ask questions and offer feedback.**
   At this time, the PI and research staff will be encouraged to share feedback about the review experience and to offer any opinions and ideas regarding research at [insert institution] in general.

Final Report and PI Response

1. **Within 2 weeks, FINAL REPORT and PI RESPONSE FORM**
   After the final meeting, the auditor will incorporate any changes to the report based on clarifications and discussion provided by the PI and research staff and will be sent out within 2 weeks.
2. **PI Response to Final Report**
   Once the PI has reviewed the report, all Required Corrective Actions must be addressed, and Recommended Actions considered. The PI

must complete, sign, and return the PI Response Form within 1 month of receipt, unless more time is requested and approved. The Response Form allows the PI to explain what actions were taken, and to explain why certain recommended actions were not implemented.

3. **PI Responses Reviewed**

   Once the QA/QI office receives the signed PI Response Form, the auditor will review the responses to ensure all actions were adequately addressed. If any issues are still unresolved, the auditor will contact the PI to ask for clarifications or to request further resolution.

4. **QA/QI Review Approved and Closed**

   Once all actions were adequately addressed, the review will be formally closed. The report will be kept confidential and will not be shared with any other departments without PI permission and/or notification.

A Note on Confidentiality of the Final Report and PI Responses

Any observations made by the auditor, the Final Report, and PI Responses will be kept CONFIDENTIAL and will not be shared with the IRB unless serious or continuing noncompliance is noted; or if a PI repeatedly fails to adequately address corrective actions required by regulations and [insert institution] policies. In both cases, the PI will be informed prior to IRB notification. The report will not be shared with any other individuals unless the PI requests.

Questions and Contact Information

If you have any questions about this process, please contact:
[insert contact information including name, phone, e-mail]

Observation Index
REGULATORY

Observation	Applicable Regulatory or Guidance Citation	Corrective Action / Best Practice Recommendation
Research Protocol is not on file.	ICH GCP 8.2.2	**Example:**
		Corrective Action: *Obtain current and previous versions of the research protocol and file appropriately in Regulatory Binder.*
		Best Practice Recommendation: *File all research protocols in reverse chronological order. Identify a member of study staff to review the Regulatory Binder to ensure completeness and accuracy.*
CVs for all study staff are not on file. CVs for all study staff are not signed and dated.	ICH-GCP 8.2.10 ICH-GCP 8.3.5 ICH-GCP 4.1.1 21 CFR 312.53(a); (c)(2) 21 CFR 812.43 (a)	**Corrective Action:** **Best Practice Recommendations:**
Current/Valid licensures are not on file.	ICH-GCP 4.1.1 ICH GCP 8.2.10 21 CFR 312.53(a) 21 CFR 812.43(a)	**Corrective Action:** **Best Practice Recommendations:**
The Screening & Enrollment Log is incomplete / not on file.	ICH-GCP 8.3.22	**Corrective Actions:** **Best Practice Recommendation:**
A Staff Signature and Delegation of Responsibility Log is incomplete / not on file.	ICH-GCP 4.1.5	**Corrective Actions:** **Best Practice Recommendation:**
The PI has not properly documented the delegation of the study tasks.	ICH-GCP 4.1.5	**Corrective Actions:** **Best Practice Recommendation:**
The Monitoring Log is incomplete / not on file.	ICH-GCP 8.3.10	**Corrective Actions:** **Best Practice Recommendation:**
Copies of all signed and dated IRB correspondences are incomplete / not on file.	ICH-GCP 4.4.1 ICH-GCP 8.3.3 ICH-GCP 8.3.11	**Corrective Actions:** **Best Practice Recommendation:**
Lab documentation is incomplete / not on file.	ICH-GCP 8.2.11 ICH-GCP 8.2.12	**Corrective Actions:** **Best Practice Recommendation:**
Valid human research training documentation is incomplete / not on file for current study staff.	ICH-GCP 4.1.1	**Corrective Actions:** **Best Practice Recommendation:**

REGULATORY (*continued*)

Observation	Applicable Regulatory or Guidance Citation	Corrective Action / Best Practice Recommendation
A Regulatory Binder is not on file.	ICH-GCP 4.9.4	Corrective Actions: Best Practice Recommendation:
Sections of the Regulatory Binder are empty.	ICH-GCP 4.9.4	Corrective Actions: Best Practice Recommendation:
Essential regulatory documentation is not adequately maintained.	ICH-GCP 4.9.4	Corrective Actions: Best Practice Recommendation:
The current Form FDA 1572 is incomplete / not on file.	21 CFR 312.53(c)(1)(i-viii)	Corrective Actions: Best Practice Recommendation:
The FDA annual report/s is/are not on file.	21 CFR 312.33 21 CFR 812.50(b)(5)	Corrective Actions: Best Practice Recommendation:
Data Safety Monitoring Board (DSMB) reports are incomplete / not on file.	ICH-GCP 5.18.6 ICH-GCP 8.3.10	Corrective Actions: Best Practice Recommendation:
Sponsor documentation is incomplete / not on file.	ICH-GCP 8.3.11 ICH-GCP 5.1.1	Corrective Actions: Best Practice Recommendation:
Documents maintained on site **[and implemented in the field]** were not submitted and approved by the IRB prior to implementation.	ICH-GCP 4.4.3	Corrective Actions: Best Practice Recommendation:
Regulatory documentation could be further streamlined.	ICH-GCP 4.9.1	Corrective Actions: Best Practice Recommendation:
The Investigator Brochure is not on file.	21 CFR 312.23(a)(5); 312.55	Corrective Actions: Best Practice Recommendation:
The Drug Accountability Log is incomplete / not on file.	21 CFR 312.57	Corrective Actions: Best Practice Recommendation:
The Device Accountability Log is incomplete / not on file.	21 CFR 812.140(b)(2)	Corrective Actions: Best Practice Recommendation:

INFORMED CONSENT

Observation	Applicable Regulatory or Guidance Citation	Corrective Action / Best Practice Recommendation
Participant ID is not on all the pages of the informed consent document.	ICH-GCP 4.9.1	**Example:** **Corrective Actions:** *Review all consent forms and place missing IDs on all pages of the consent form for every identified participant.* **Best Practice Recommendation:** *Identify a member of the study staff to review informed consent form documentation regularly for errors and omissions and to ensure completeness.*
Informed consent was not appropriately documented. (e.g., The participant and/or study representative signed on the wrong line.)	ICH-GCP 4.8.9	**Corrective Actions:** **Best Practice Recommendation:**
The options section(s) located within the text of the consent form are incomplete.	ICH-GCP 4.9.1	**Corrective Actions:** **Best Practice Recommendation:**
Informed consent wasn't obtained and/or not documented without an IRB-approved waiver.	45 CFR 46.117(c) 21 CFR 50.23	**Corrective Actions:** **Best Practice Recommendation:**
Dating discrepancies were found between the participant and study representative.	ICH-GCP 4.9.1	**Corrective Actions:** **Best Practice Recommendation:**
A minor was enrolled without obtaining parental permission as required in the IRB-approved protocol.	45 CFR 46.408 21 CFR 50.55	**Corrective Actions:** **Best Practice Recommendation:**
Witness signatures are inconsistently documented on the consent form. The protocol does not require a witness signature.	45 CFR 46.117(b)(2) ICH-GCP 4.8.9 21 CFR 50.27(b)(2)	**Corrective Actions:** **Best Practice Recommendation:**
The re-consenting process was not adequately conducted for all participants.	ICH-GCP 4.8.2	**Corrective Actions:** **Best Practice Recommendation:**
A copy of the consent form was not given to the participant(s).	45 CFR 46.117 21 CFR 50.27(a)	**Corrective Actions:** **Best Practice Recommendation:**

INFORMED CONSENT (*continued*)

Observation	Applicable Regulatory or Guidance Citation	Corrective Action / Best Practice Recommendation
Informed consent was not adequately obtained for all participants. Participant signatures and/or dates are not documented on all consent forms.	45 CFR 46.117 ICH-GCP 4.8.8 21 CFR 50.20 21 CFR 812.140(a)(3)(i)	Corrective Actions: Best Practice Recommendation:
An English consent form was used to obtain consent from a non-English speaking participant(s).	45 CFR 46.117(b)(2) 45 CFR 46.116 21 CFR 50.20	Corrective Actions: Best Practice Recommendation:
A consent form is not on file for all participants.	45 CFR 312.62(b) 21 CFR 46.116	Corrective Actions: Best Practice Recommendation:
Invalid, outdated consent forms were used to consent participants.	45 CFR 46.116 ICH-GCP 4.8.1	Corrective Actions: Best Practice Recommendation:
Original consent forms are not on file for participants enrolled in the study.	45 CFR 46.117 ICH-GCP 4.8.11	Corrective Actions: Best Practice Recommendation:
Participants signed consent and were enrolled into the study during a lapse of IRB approval.	45 CFR 46 21 CFR 312.66	Corrective Actions: Best Practice Recommendation:

PARTICIPANT FILES

Observation	Applicable Regulatory or Guidance Citation	Corrective Action / Best Practice Recommendation
Study documentation has been inappropriately obscured.	ICH-GCP 4.9.3	**Example:** **Corrective Actions:** *Write a signed and dated Note-to-File documenting the findings.* **Best Practice Recommendation:** *Corrections should be made using a single-line cross-out to ensure that the correction being made does not obscure the original entry. The person making the correction should initial and date the revision.*
Dating discrepancies were observed in source documentation.	ICH-GCP 4.9.1	**Corrective Actions:** **Best Practice Recommendation:**
Blank fields and incomplete data entries were observed throughout the participant's files.	ICH-GCP 4.9.1 21 CFR 312.62(b)	**Corrective Actions:** **Best Practice Recommendation:**
There are no comments on file regarding the clinical significance of out-of-range/flagged lab values.	ICH-GCP 4.3.2	**Corrective Actions:** **Best Practice Recommendation:**
The clinician's signature is missing on assessments.	ICH GCP 8.3.14	**Corrective Actions:** **Best Practice Recommendation:**
Source documentation to verify eligibility is not on file.	ICH-GCP 8.3.13 21 CFR 312.62(b) 21 CFR 812.140(a)(3)(i-iii)	**Corrective Actions:** **Best Practice Recommendation:**
Exceptions to inclusion/exclusion criteria have been made for participants. No IRB documentation to confirm approval of exceptions.	ICH-GCP 4.5.2 21 CFR 312.60 21 CFR 312.66	**Corrective Actions:** **Best Practice Recommendation:**
Source documents / participant documentation forms are not signed and dated by the person performing the exam.	ICH-GCP 8.3.14 21 CFR 312.62(b) 21 CFR 812.140(a)(3)(i-iii)	**Corrective Actions:** **Best Practice Recommendation:**
Study procedures were not done according to the IRB-approved protocol.	ICH-GCP 4.5.2 21 CFR 312.60 21 CFR 312.66 21 CFR 812.140(a)(4)	**Corrective Actions:** **Best Practice Recommendation:**

PARTICIPANT FILES (*continued*)

Observation	Applicable Regulatory or Guidance Citation	Corrective Action / Best Practice Recommendation
Reportable Information identified during the Quality Improvement Program review of the participant's files. Documentation indicating the PI's assessment and reporting of these findings is not on file.	**ICH-GCP 4.11.1** **21 CFR 312.64(b)** **21 CFR 812.140(b)(5)**	**Corrective Actions:** **Best Practice Recommendation:**
Participant files are not well organized.	**ICH-GCP 4.9.1**	**Corrective Actions:** **Best Practice Recommendation:**

Model Audit Tool

INSTRUCTIONS FOR MODEL AUDIT TOOL

This comprehensive tool may be used to record information at time of review. Check each item as it is reviewed and completed and record pertinent comments.

For certain studies, some of the data on the audit tool may not be applicable and the auditor may mark the "N/A" checkbox. There is space to write down any notes or additional comments after each section.

This audit tool is a template and can be modified and adapted according to your institution's needs. Refer to your institution's regulations, policies, and/or guidance documents for further clarification of what is required.

MODEL AUDIT TOOL   Interview Questions

Interview Segments Covered (use as a cover sheet to indicate segments covered in the interview)
Please complete relevant questions from the list below.

Protocol Number: _____   **Interview Date:** _____

Interview Segments Covered	N/A	Yes	No
1. Study Staff	☐	☐	☐
a. Staff Training	☐	☐	☐
2. Study Teams SOPs	☐	☐	☐
3. Subject Participation	☐	☐	☐
a. Recruitment process	☐	☐	☐
b. Consenting process (who consents subjects, where, when)	☐	☐	☐
c. Data Collection / Study Visits	☐	☐	☐
4. Study materials - Storage	☐	☐	☐
5. Data notebooks	☐	☐	☐
6. Electronic data storage	☐	☐	☐
7. Missing data	☐	☐	☐
8. Drug/Device Accountability	☐	☐	☐
9. Staff communication system	☐	☐	☐
10. Study meetings	☐	☐	☐
11. Communication and handling of study problems including protocol deviations, and adverse and unanticipated events	☐	☐	☐
12. Adequate resources and staff to conduct study? Staff turnovers?	☐	☐	☐
13. Participant safety and data monitoring (outside monitoring, DSMB)	☐	☐	☐
14. Delays in IRB submissions, temporary terminations	☐	☐	☐
15. Obstacles to conducting research	☐	☐	☐
16. Suggested Improvements to facilitate research	☐	☐	☐

Notes or Additional Comments:

A. Study Personnel

Protocol Number: _____ Interview Date: _____		Information obtained during Interview*			
Role	**Name**	**Subj**	**IC**	**Data**	**Present**
Principal Investigator		☐	☐	☐	☐
Co-PI (if applicable)		☐	☐	☐	☐
Co-Investigators		☐	☐	☐	☐
		☐	☐	☐	☐
		☐	☐	☐	☐
		☐	☐	☐	☐
		☐	☐	☐	☐
		☐	☐	☐	☐
Project Coordinator		☐	☐	☐	☐
Research Assistants		☐	☐	☐	☐
		☐	☐	☐	☐
		☐	☐	☐	☐
		☐	☐	☐	☐
		☐	☐	☐	☐
		☐	☐	☐	☐
		☐	☐	☐	☐
Consultants		☐	☐	☐	☐
		☐	☐	☐	☐
		☐	☐	☐	☐
Statisticians		☐	☐	☐	☐
		☐	☐	☐	☐
		☐	☐	☐	☐
		☐	☐	☐	☐
		☐	☐	☐	☐
Other:		☐	☐	☐	☐
		☐	☐	☐	☐
		☐	☐	☐	☐
		☐	☐	☐	☐

* Interview Information: Subj = Contact with Subjects; IC = Involved with Informed Consent process; Data = Contact with Data; Present = Present at Interview

B. Interview Questions

1. Describe the current study organization: (i.e., Who is involved? What is everyone's responsibility?)

   a. How is study staff trained?

   b. Is there documentation of completion of study specific training?   ☐ Yes   ☐ No

   c. Who is responsible for preparing IRB Amendment Applications?

      Name: _____   Role: _____

   d. Who is responsible for preparing IRB Continuing Review Applications?

      Name: _____   Role: _____

   e. Who is responsible for preparing AEs, UPs, or other reportable information?

      Name: _____   Role: _____

2. Are there Study SOPs?   ☐ Yes   ☐ No

   a. Where are they kept and who is responsible for updating them?

3. Walk through a subject's participation in the study from recruitment to endpoint.

   a. Recruitment process:

      i. How are subjects identified?

      ii. Are subjects pre-screened prior to enrollment?   ☐ Yes   ☐ No

      iii. How are subjects reviewed/screened for eligibility?

      iv. Who makes initial contact with subjects?

         Name: _____   Role: _____

         Name: _____   Role: _____

         Name: _____   Role: _____

      v. How is initial contact made?

→ ☐ *Are procedures implemented as written in the approved protocol?*

b. Consent process:

    i. Who consents participants?

    Name: _____   Role: _____

    Name: _____   Role: _____

    Name: _____   Role: _____

    ii. Where are subjects consented?

    iii. When are subjects consented?

→ ☐ *Are procedures implemented as written in the approved protocol?*

Do subjects/guardians receive a copy of the consent?	☐ Yes	☐ No	☐ N/A
Are consents filed in medical records?	☐ Yes	☐ No	☐ N/A

What other research information (if any) is filed in medical records?

c. Data Collection / Study Visits

→ ☐ *Are procedures implemented as written in the approved protocol?*

4. Where and how are study materials stored? (i.e., Who has access to location? Locked?)

→ ☐ *Are procedures implemented as written in the approved protocol?*

5. Are there lab/data notebooks?	☐ Yes	☐ No	☐ N/A

    a. If yes, are they paper, electronic, or both?

      ☐ Paper   ☐ Electronic

    b. Who has access to the data – both paper and electronic?

c. Is there a Data Coordinating Center?	☐ Yes	☐ No

6. How is electronic data stored? (i.e., Is there a single database, multiple databases? Who enters the data? Who makes or authorizes changes in the database? Who runs analyses? Who has access to the electronic records?)

7. Do you have an SOP for handling missing data?   ☐ Yes   ☐ No

→ ☐ *Note: If yes, Review SOP during Data Security/Confidentiality Portion of PI Review*

   a. If no, can you describe what you would do if you discovered data was missing?

8. How is study drug/device accountability handled? (i.e., How dispensed? By whom?)

   a. How is documentation of dispensing done?

9. Is there a good communication system between the PI(s) and the research staff? (i.e., How are changes in protocol communicated? Problems with recruiting, problems with data collection, etc.?)

10. Is there a weekly or regular meeting to discuss the study? (i.e., Progress, process of data collection, quality of data collected, what the data looks like, or what it indicates so far)

   a. Who attends these meetings? (intended to ascertain if PI is actively involved in study)

   b. Do you keep minutes of team meetings?   ☐ Yes   ☐ No

   c. Are they kept in the regulatory binder or other centralized location accessible to study   ☐ Yes   ☐ No
     staff?

11. How are protocol problems, deviations, adverse and unanticipated events communicated to the PI and other study personnel? (intended to ascertain communication within study re: important events)

→ ☐ *Note: Review what is serious, what might be an unanticipated event, and what might be an adverse event.*

   a. How are protocol problems, deviations, adverse and unanticipated events documented and reported? (intended to ascertain if there is a systematic way that the site captures and reports events)

12. Are there adequate resources and staff to conduct this study? (i.e., Staff turnover?)

13. How is participant safety and data protection monitored?

    a. Is there a Data Monitoring Plan (DSMP)?   ☐ Yes   ☐ No

    b. Is there a Data Monitoring Board (DSMB)?   ☐ Yes   ☐ No

       If yes, when was the last meeting of the DSMB?

    c. Has there been any other outside monitoring of the study?   ☐ Yes   ☐ No

       If yes, by whom, what date, and for what reason?

→ ☐ *Note: All such outside reports should be submitted to the IRB*

14. Please explain any abnormally long delays in IRB submissions (if applicable):

15. Are there any obstacles to conducting this study here at [*institution*]?

16. What would be most helpful for you when conducting research at [*institution*]?

Additional Interview Notes:

MODEL AUDIT TOOL   Auditor Observations

This is a model audit tool. Depending upon internal processes, information may be reviewed at different times during the preparation for or conduct of an audit. Please feel free to modify this tool so that it is appropriate for use at your institution.

1. Documentation		IRB Review			PI Review		
a. *Initial Approval*		N/A or N/R*	Yes	No	N/A or N/R*	Yes	No
A copy of the current protocol is on file		☐	☐	☐	☐	☐	☐
A copy of the grant, contract, or funding application is on file			☐	☐		☐	☐
The Initial Application is appropriately signed and dated			☐	☐		☐	☐
All additional forms required for the initial approval are on-file		☐	☐	☐	☐	☐	☐
Approved recruitment materials are on file	Number: ____	☐	☐	☐	☐	☐	☐
Approved informed consent forms are on file	Number: ____	☐	☐	☐	☐	☐	☐
Approved assent forms are on file	Number: ____	☐	☐	☐	☐	☐	☐
Approved data collection instruments are on file	Number: ____	☐	☐	☐	☐	☐	☐
Approved flow charts and/or schemas are on file	Number: ____	☐	☐	☐	☐	☐	☐
Approved study documents are on file (reminders, thank yous, etc)	Number: ____	☐	☐	☐	☐	☐	☐
The Initial Approval letter is on file			☐	☐		☐	☐

Notes:

Documentation (continued)	IRB Review			PI Review		
b. *Amendments*	N/A or N/R*	Yes	No	N/A or N/R*	Yes	No
There have been amendments to the protocol Number: _____		☐	☐		☐	☐
Amendment #_____ Application for this amendment is on file	☐	☐	☐	☐	☐	☐
Amendment content:						
Supplementary materials were approved as part of amendment		☐	☐		☐	☐
Amendment involved changes to the consent form		☐	☐		☐	☐
If yes, please specify:						
Approval Letter is on file Approval Date: _____						
Amendment #_____ Application for this amendment is on file	☐	☐	☐	☐	☐	☐
Amendment content:						
Supplementary materials were approved as part of amendment		☐	☐		☐	☐
Amendment involved changes to the consent form		☐	☐		☐	☐
If yes, please specify:						
Approval Letter is on file Approval Date: _____						
Amendment #_____ Application for this amendment is on file	☐	☐	☐	☐	☐	☐
Amendment content:						
Supplementary materials were approved as part of amendment		☐	☐		☐	☐
Amendment involved changes to the consent form		☐	☐		☐	☐
If yes, please specify:						
Approval Letter is on file Approval Date: _____						
Amendment #_____ Application for this amendment is on file	☐	☐	☐	☐	☐	☐
Amendment content:						
Supplementary materials were approved as part of amendment		☐	☐		☐	☐
Amendment involved changes to the consent form		☐	☐		☐	☐
If yes, please specify:						
Approval Letter is on file Approval Date: _____						
Amendment #_____ Application for this amendment is on file	☐	☐	☐	☐	☐	☐
Amendment content:						
Supplementary materials were approved as part of amendment		☐	☐		☐	☐
Amendment involved changes to the consent form		☐	☐		☐	☐
If yes, please specify:						
Approval Letter is on file Approval Date: _____						

Documentation (continued)	IRB Review			PI Review		
c. *Continuing Reviews*	N/A or N/R*	Yes	No	N/A or N/R*	Yes	No
There have been Continuing Reviews (CR) Number: _____	☐	☐	☐	☐	☐	☐
CR #_____ Application for this CR is on file		☐	☐		☐	☐
Approval Letter is on file Approval Date: _____						
CR #_____ Application for this CR is on file		☐	☐		☐	☐
Approval Letter is on file Approval Date: _____						
CR #_____ Application for this CR is on file		☐	☐		☐	☐
Approval Letter is on file Approval Date: _____						
CR #_____ Application for this CR is on file		☐	☐		☐	☐
Approval Letter is on file Approval Date: _____						
CR #_____ Application for this CR is on file		☐	☐		☐	☐
Approval Letter is on file Approval Date: _____						
CR #_____ Application for this CR is on file		☐	☐		☐	☐
Approval Letter is on file Approval Date: _____						
There was a lapse period between any protocol expiration date and the CR approval (CR #_____)	☐	☐	☐	☐	☐	☐
If Yes — Were any subjects enrolled during the lapse period?	☐	☐	☐	☐	☐	☐
If Yes — Was a protocol violation form submitted to the IRB?	☐	☐	☐	☐	☐	☐
If Yes — Were any study procedures done during the lapse period?	☐	☐	☐	☐	☐	☐
If Yes — Were the procedures done during the lapse period approved by the IRB?	☐	☐	☐	☐	☐	☐
A copy of the most recent NIH or Sponsor Progress Report is on file	☐	☐	☐	☐	☐	☐
All correspondence with the IRB is on file	☐	☐	☐	☐	☐	☐

Notes:

Documentation (continued)		IRB Review			PI Review		
d. *Review of Additional Sites / External IRB Approvals*		N/A or N/R*	Yes	No	N/A or N/R*	Yes	No
The IRB is responsible for the review of additional sites	Number: ____		☐	☐		☐	☐
Name:	FWA: _____						
Location:							
Current (unexpired) approval letter is on file	Date: _____	☐	☐	☐	☐	☐	☐
Name:	FWA: _____						
Location:							
Current (unexpired) approval letter is on file	Date: _____	☐	☐	☐	☐	☐	☐
Name:	FWA: _____						
Location:							
Current (unexpired) approval letter is on file	Date: _____	☐	☐	☐	☐	☐	☐
Name:	FWA: _____						
Location:							
Current (unexpired) approval letter is on file	Date: _____	☐	☐	☐	☐	☐	☐
Name:	FWA: _____						
Location:							
Current (unexpired) approval letter is on file	Date: _____	☐	☐	☐	☐	☐	☐
There are external IRB approvals	Number: ____						
Name:	FWA: _____						
Location:							
Current (unexpired) approval letter is on file	Date: _____	☐	☐	☐	☐	☐	☐
Name:	FWA: _____						
Location:							
Current (unexpired) approval letter is on file	Date: _____	☐	☐	☐	☐	☐	☐
Name:	FWA: _____						
Location:							
Current (unexpired) approval letter is on file	Date: _____	☐	☐	☐	☐	☐	☐
Name: _____	FWA: _____						
Location: _____							
Current (unexpired) approval letter is on file	Date: _____	☐	☐	☐	☐	☐	☐

2. Regulatory Documentation			IRB Review			PI Review		
			N/A or N/R*	Yes	No	N/A or N/R*	Yes	No
This is an FDA regulated study				☐	☐		☐	☐
If Yes		FDA 1572 is current, signed and dated	☐	☐	☐	☐	☐	☐
		The Clinical Investigator Financial Disclosure form is on file for each investigator (*FDA 3455 or 3454*)		☐	☐		☐	☐
		The PI is an IND/IDE holder	☐	☐	☐	☐	☐	☐
	If Yes	Original FDA 1571 (IND only) is current, signed, dated		☐	☐		☐	☐
		FDA 1571 is on file for all amendments		☐	☐		☐	☐
		FDA 1571 is on file for all Annual and Safety Reports		☐	☐		☐	☐
		Name of Monitor listed in section 14 of most recent FDA 1571:						
Lab certifications are on file			☐	☐	☐	☐	☐	☐
Lab normal values are on file						☐	☐	☐
Lab Director's CV is on file						☐	☐	☐
Investigator Brochure and package inserts are on file						☐	☐	☐
Current SOPs or MOO is on file						☐	☐	☐
Monitoring Log is up to date						☐	☐	☐
Currently approved Case Report Forms are on file						☐	☐	☐
Currently approved Source Documents are on file (Source Log)						☐	☐	☐
Roles and Responsibilities Log is up to date						☐	☐	☐
Staff Signature Log is up to date						☐	☐	☐
All correspondence to and from the sponsor if on file						☐	☐	☐

Notes:

3. Drug/Device Dispensing Accountability	IRB Review			PI Review		
	N/A or N/R*	Yes	No	N/A or N/R*	Yes	No
Drugs or devices are used in this study protocol		☐	☐		☐	☐
Documentation of drug/device use for each subject is available		☐	☐		☐	☐
A dispensing and accountability log is maintained	☐	☐	☐	☐	☐	☐
The log includes all necessary elements	☐	☐	☐	☐	☐	☐
Protocol identifier	☐	☐	☐	☐	☐	☐
Subject identifier	☐	☐	☐	☐	☐	☐
Randomization # or Kit #	☐	☐	☐	☐	☐	☐
Initials of person dispensing/receiving	☐	☐	☐	☐	☐	☐
Date dispensed	☐	☐	☐	☐	☐	☐
Amount dispensed	☐	☐	☐	☐	☐	☐
Date returned	☐	☐	☐	☐	☐	☐
Amount returned	☐	☐	☐	☐	☐	☐
The drug dose is being administered and used as approved	☐	☐	☐	☐	☐	☐
Shipping/receiving is handled by: ☐ Study site ☐ Research Pharmacy ☐ Other:						
Shipping/receiving receipts are on file		☐	☐		☐	☐
Appropriate documentation for the return/destruction of unused drugs/devices is available		☐	☐		☐	☐

The "If Yes" labels (outer and inner) apply to the grouped rows: the outer "If Yes" spans from "Documentation of drug/device use..." through "Appropriate documentation...", and the inner "If Yes" spans the log element rows ("The log includes all necessary elements" through "Amount returned").

Notes:

4. Monitoring	IRB Review			PI Review		
	N/A or N/R*	Yes	No	N/A or N/R*	Yes	No
This study requires a Data Safety Monitoring Plan (DSMP)		☐	☐		☐	☐
If Yes — The DSMP includes the 4 basic features		☐	☐		☐	☐
Process to monitor research progress for patient safety		☐	☐		☐	☐
Process of detecting and reporting adverse events (AEs)		☐	☐		☐	☐
Process of reporting actions resulting in study suspension to the PI, Sponsor and IRB in a timely fashion		☐	☐		☐	☐
Process for assuring data accuracy & protocol compliance		☐	☐		☐	☐
A copy of the DSMP is on file		☐	☐		☐	☐
This study has a Data Monitoring Board (DSMB)		☐	☐		☐	☐
If Yes — Members of the DSMB are independent (*not related to study conduct or interests*)		☐	☐		☐	☐
If sponsored research, at least one member of the DSMB is independent of the company		☐	☐		☐	☐
Members of the DSMB have adequate expertise		☐	☐		☐	☐
The DSMB has met in accordance with the IRB approved protocol		☐	☐		☐	☐
All DSMB reports are on file		☐	☐		☐	☐
This study has had other monitoring (*by sponsor, institution, QA/QI*)		☐	☐		☐	☐
If Yes — Monitoring group:		☐	☐		☐	☐
Report is on file Monitoring Date:		☐	☐		☐	☐
All items that require IRB notification have been submitted		☐	☐		☐	☐
All outstanding issues from the Monitoring Report have been addressed		☐	☐		☐	☐
Monitoring group:		☐	☐		☐	☐
Report is on file Monitoring Date:		☐	☐		☐	☐
All items that require IRB notification have been submitted		☐	☐		☐	☐
All outstanding issues from the Monitoring Report have been addressed		☐	☐		☐	☐
Monitoring group:		☐	☐		☐	☐
Report is on file Monitoring Date:		☐	☐		☐	☐
All items that require IRB notification have been submitted		☐	☐		☐	☐
All outstanding issues from the Monitoring Report have been addressed		☐	☐		☐	☐

5. Adverse Events / Unexpected Problems	IRB Review			PI Review		
a. Local Events	N/A or N/R*	Yes	No	N/A or N/R*	Yes	No
Internal Adverse Events (AEs) have Number: _____ occurred (*use additional form to report AEs if necessary*)		☐	☐		☐	☐
Date of event: _____ ☐ Serious ☐ Unexpected Date reported to IRB: _____ ☐ Other: Description: IRB action: Event was reported to DSMB, FDA, &/or sponsor (*as applicable*)	☐	☐	☐	☐	☐	☐
Date of event: _____ ☐ Serious ☐ Unexpected Date reported to IRB: _____ ☐ Other: Description: IRB action: Event was reported to DSMB, FDA, &/or sponsor (*as applicable*)	☐	☐	☐	☐	☐	☐
Date of event: _____ ☐ Serious ☐ Unexpected Date reported to IRB: _____ ☐ Other: Description: IRB action: Event was reported to DSMB, FDA, &/or sponsor (*as applicable*)	☐	☐	☐	☐	☐	☐
Date of event: _____ ☐ Serious ☐ Unexpected Date reported to IRB: _____ ☐ Other: Description: IRB action: Event was reported to DSMB, FDA, &/or sponsor (*as applicable*)	☐	☐	☐	☐	☐	☐

If Yes (applies to the rows above)

Notes:

e. Adverse Events / Unexpected Problems (continued)	IRB Review			PI Review		
a. Local Events (continued)	N/A or N/R*	Yes	No	N/A or N/R*	Yes	No
Internal Unexpected Problems (UPs) Number: _____ have occurred (*use additional form to report UPs if necessary*)		☐	☐		☐	☐
Date of event: _____ ☐ Serious Date reported to IRB: _____ ☐ Other: Description: IRB action: Event was reported to DSMB, FDA, &/or sponsor (*as applicable*)	☐	☐	☐	☐	☐	☐
Date of event: _____ ☐ Serious Date reported to IRB: _____ ☐ Other: Description: IRB action: Event was reported to DSMB, FDA, &/or sponsor (*as applicable*)	☐	☐	☐	☐	☐	☐
Date of event: _____ ☐ Serious Date reported to IRB: _____ ☐ Other: Description: IRB action: Event was reported to DSMB, FDA, &/or sponsor (*as applicable*)	☐	☐	☐	☐	☐	☐
Date of event: _____ ☐ Serious Date reported to IRB: _____ ☐ Other: Description: IRB action: Event was reported to DSMB, FDA, &/or sponsor (*as applicable*)	☐	☐	☐	☐	☐	☐

If Yes

Notes:

5. Adverse Events / Unexpected Problems (continued)	IRB Review			PI Review		
a. Off-Site Events	N/A or N/R*	Yes	No	N/A or N/R*	Yes	No
Off-site Adverse Events (AEs) have Number: ___ occurred (*use additional form to report AEs if necessary*)		☐	☐		☐	☐
If Yes — Date of event: _____ ☐ Serious ☐ Unexpected / Date reported to IRB: _____ ☐ Other: / Description: / IRB action: / Event was reported to DSMB, FDA, &/or sponsor (*as applicable*)	☐	☐	☐	☐	☐	☐
Date of event: _____ ☐ Serious ☐ Unexpected / Date reported to IRB: _____ ☐ Other: / Description: / IRB action: / Event was reported to DSMB, FDA, &/or sponsor (*as applicable*)	☐	☐	☐	☐	☐	☐
Off-site Unexpected Problems (UPs) Number: ___ have occurred (*use additional form to report UPs if necessary*)		☐	☐		☐	☐
If Yes — Date of event: _____ ☐ Serious / Date reported to IRB: _____ ☐ Other: / Description: / IRB action: / Event was reported to DSMB, FDA, &/or sponsor (*as applicable*)	☐	☐	☐	☐	☐	☐
Date of event: _____ ☐ Serious / Date reported to IRB: _____ ☐ Other: / Description: / IRB action: / Event was reported to DSMB, FDA, &/or sponsor (*as applicable*)	☐	☐	☐	☐	☐	☐
All AE and UP reports, IRB submissions and IRB responses are on file		☐	☐		☐	☐

Notes:

6. Protocol Violations/Deviations / Noncompliance	IRB Review			PI Review		
	N/A or N/R*	Yes	No	N/A or N/R*	Yes	No
Protocol violations/deviations have Number: ____ occurred (*use additional form to report violations/deviations if necessary*)		☐	☐			
If Yes — Date of event: _____ ☐ Minor Date reported to IRB: _____ ☐ Significant Description: IRB action: Event was reported to DSMB, FDA, &/or sponsor (*as applicable*)	☐	☐	☐	☐		
Date of event: _____ ☐ Minor Date reported to IRB: _____ ☐ Significant Description: IRB action: Event was reported to DSMB, FDA, &/or sponsor (*as applicable*)	☐	☐	☐	☐		
Date of event: _____ ☐ Minor Date reported to IRB: ____ ☐ Significant Description: IRB action: Event was reported to DSMB, FDA, &/or sponsor (*as applicable*)	☐	☐	☐	☐		
For each deviation / incident of noncompliance there was adequate follow up and resolution		☐	☐	☐		
All deviations / incidents of noncompliance were reported to the IRB		☐	☐	☐		
All deviations / incident reports, IRB submissions, and IRB responses are on file		☐	☐	☐		

Notes:

MODEL AUDIT TOOL   Regulatory

This is a model audit tool. Depending upon internal processes, information may be reviewed at different times during the preparation for or conduct of an audit. Please feel free to modify this tool so that it is appropriate for use at your institution.

General Information   Protocol Number: _____

PI Last Name: PI First Name:

Responsible Institution: Ceded Review Institution:

Department:

Study Title:

Funding Source / Grant Number: _____

Funding	☐ None	☐ Internal/Department	☐ Industry
	☐ Government	☐ Foundation	☐ Other

Date of Initial IRB Approval: _____   Current Expiration Date: _____

QA Review

Name of QA Reviewer: _____   QA Reviewer's Institution: _____

Selection Type	☐ Not For Cause – Random	☐ For Cause
	☐ Not For Cause – Requested by _____ Date Requested: _____	

Date of Review: _____

A. Study Personnel				Obtained during review of Regulatory Documents						
Protocol Number: _____	CV information			Research		Additional Training / Licensure				
Name All Study Staff	CV	2yr	sign	Hum subj	COI	Med	Lab	Phleb	Other 1	Other 2
Principal Investigator	☐	☐	☐	☐	☐	☐	☐	☐	☐	☐
Co-PI (if applicable)	☐	☐	☐	☐	☐	☐	☐	☐	☐	☐
Co-Investigators	☐	☐	☐	☐	☐	☐	☐	☐	☐	☐
	☐	☐	☐	☐	☐	☐	☐	☐	☐	☐
	☐	☐	☐	☐	☐	☐	☐	☐	☐	☐
	☐	☐	☐	☐	☐	☐	☐	☐	☐	☐
	☐	☐	☐	☐	☐	☐	☐	☐	☐	☐
	☐	☐	☐	☐	☐	☐	☐	☐	☐	☐
	☐	☐	☐	☐	☐	☐	☐	☐	☐	☐

	CV information			Research		Additional Training / Licensure				
Name All Study Staff	CV	2yr	sign	Hum subj	COI	Med	Lab	Phleb	Other 1	Other 2
Project Coordinator	☐	☐	☐	☐	☐	☐	☐	☐	☐	☐
Research Assistants	☐	☐	☐	☐	☐	☐	☐	☐	☐	☐
	☐	☐	☐	☐	☐	☐	☐	☐	☐	☐
	☐	☐	☐	☐	☐	☐	☐	☐	☐	☐
	☐	☐	☐	☐	☐	☐	☐	☐	☐	☐
	☐	☐	☐	☐	☐	☐	☐	☐	☐	☐
	☐	☐	☐	☐	☐	☐	☐	☐	☐	☐
	☐	☐	☐	☐	☐	☐	☐	☐	☐	☐
Consultants	☐	☐	☐	☐	☐	☐	☐	☐	☐	☐
	☐	☐	☐	☐	☐	☐	☐	☐	☐	☐
	☐	☐	☐	☐	☐	☐	☐	☐	☐	☐
	☐	☐	☐	☐	☐	☐	☐	☐	☐	☐
	☐	☐	☐	☐	☐	☐	☐	☐	☐	☐
	☐	☐	☐	☐	☐	☐	☐	☐	☐	☐
Statisticians	☐	☐	☐	☐	☐	☐	☐	☐	☐	☐
	☐	☐	☐	☐	☐	☐	☐	☐	☐	☐
	☐	☐	☐	☐	☐	☐	☐	☐	☐	☐
	☐	☐	☐	☐	☐	☐	☐	☐	☐	☐
	☐	☐	☐	☐	☐	☐	☐	☐	☐	☐
Other Researchers	☐	☐	☐	☐	☐	☐	☐	☐	☐	☐
	☐	☐	☐	☐	☐	☐	☐	☐	☐	☐
	☐	☐	☐	☐	☐	☐	☐	☐	☐	☐
	☐	☐	☐	☐	☐	☐	☐	☐	☐	☐
	☐	☐	☐	☐	☐	☐	☐	☐	☐	☐
	☐	☐	☐	☐	☐	☐	☐	☐	☐	☐

CV INFORMATION: CV - available for review; 2yr = CV updated within the past 2 years; Sign = CV is signed and dated
TRAINING: Hum Subj = valid (unexpired) human subjects training is on file; COI = Conflict of Interest form is on file (if applicable)
OTHER TRAINING/LICENSURE: Med = medical license is current and on file; Lab = lab safety training has been completed and certificate is on file; Phleb = phlebotomy training has been completed and certificate is on file; Other1 and Other2 = note below

Other 1:   Other 2:

B. Record Keeping   Protocol Number: _____

General Information	N/A or N/R*	Yes	No
The PI keeps a binder or folder for required IRB and regulatory documentation		☐	☐
The PI keeps a separate study file for each participant	☐	☐	☐

	IRB Review			PI Review		
7. Regulatory Documentation	N/A or N/R*	Yes	No	N/A or N/R*	Yes	No
This is an FDA regulated study		☐	☐		☐	☐
If Yes — FDA 1572 is current, signed and dated	☐	☐	☐	☐	☐	☐
The Clinical Investigator Financial Disclosure form is on file for each investigator (FDA 3455 or 3454)		☐	☐		☐	☐
The PI is an IND/IDE holder	☐	☐	☐	☐	☐	☐
If Yes — Original FDA 1571 (IND only) is current, signed, dated		☐	☐		☐	☐
FDA 1571 is on file for all amendments		☐	☐		☐	☐
FDA 1571 is on file for all Annual and Safety Reports		☐	☐		☐	☐
Name of Monitor listed in section 14 of most recent FDA 1571:						
Lab certifications are on file					☐	☐
Lab normal values are on file					☐	☐
Lab Director's CV is on file					☐	☐
Investigator Brochure and package inserts are on file					☐	☐
Current SOPs or MOO is on file					☐	☐
Monitoring Log is up to date					☐	☐
Currently approved Case Report Forms are on file					☐	☐
Currently approved Source Documents are on file (Source Log)					☐	☐
Roles and Responsibilities Log is up to date					☐	☐
Staff Signature Log is up to date					☐	☐
All correspondence to and from the sponsor is on file					☐	☐

Notes:

8. Documentation		IRB Review			PI Review	
Initial Approval	N/A or N/R*	Yes	No	N/A or N/R*	Yes	No
A copy of the current protocol is on file		☐	☐		☐	☐
A copy of the grant, contract, or funding application is on file		☐	☐		☐	☐
The Initial Application is appropriately signed and dated		☐	☐		☐	☐
All additional forms required for the initial approval are on file	☐	☐	☐	☐	☐	☐
Approved recruitment materials are on file Number: ____	☐	☐	☐	☐	☐	☐
Approved informed consent forms are on file Number: ____	☐	☐	☐	☐	☐	☐
Approved assent forms are on file Number: ____	☐	☐	☐	☐	☐	☐
Approved data collection instruments are on file Number: ____	☐	☐	☐	☐	☐	☐
Approved flow charts and/or schemas are on file Number: ____	☐	☐	☐	☐	☐	☐
Approved study documents are on file Number: ____ (*including reminders, thank yous, etc*)	☐	☐	☐	☐	☐	☐
The Initial Approval letter is on file		☐	☐		☐	☐

Notes:

		IRB Review			PI Review	
9. Consent	N/A or N/R*	Yes	No	N/A or N/R*	Yes	No
Informed consent/assent is required for this protocol		☐	☐		☐	☐

a. Waivers

		IRB Review			PI Review		
The PI requested a HIPAA Waiver/Alteration of Patient Authorization			☐	☐		☐	☐
If Yes	A copy of the approved HIPAA Waiver is on file			☐	☐		☐	☐
There is a Waiver of Consent or Documentation of Consent				☐	☐		☐	☐
If Yes	Waiver or alteration of informed consent (45 CFR 46.116(d))	☐	☐	☐	☐	☐	☐
	Waiver of documentation of informed consent (45 CFR 46.117(c))	☐	☐	☐	☐	☐	☐

b. Certificate of Confidentiality

	IRB Review			PI Review		
There is a Certificate of Confidentiality		☐	☐		☐	☐
If Yes — Certificate of Confidentiality Number: _____ Expiration Date: _____						
All (current and previous) versions of the approved and stamped consent/assent forms are on file		☐	☐		☐	☐
Invalid consents have been used		☐	☐		☐	☐
If Yes — Was the protocol deviation reported to the IRB		☐	☐		☐	☐

Number of different *active* consents or assents used for this protocol _____

Consent/Assent Title (*List title for each currently approved consent/assent*)	Version	Approval Date	Consent	Assent
			☐	☐
			☐	☐
			☐	☐
			☐	☐
			☐	☐
			☐	☐
			☐	☐

Study staff responsible for obtaining informed consent/assent

Name   Role

PI is involved in the consent process   □ Yes   □ No

	IRB Review			PI Review		
	N/A or N/R*	Yes	No	N/A or N/R*	Yes	No
The consent is in clear, understandable language		□	□		□	□
The consent is translated into other languages		□	□		□	□
If Yes There is a translation attestation on file (if applicable)		□	□		□	□
The consent/assent adequately explains all study procedures		□	□		□	□
Experimental procedures are clearly identified and explained	□	□	□	□	□	□

The consent form addresses all basic elements of informed consent**   □ Yes   □ No

Elements of Consent (** *Indicates Basic Element of Informed Consent*)

□ Research Study**
□ Purpose of Study**
□ Description of Procedures**
□ Duration of Participation**
□ Risks**
□ Benefits**
□ Alternatives**
□ Confidentiality**
□ ID of any Experimental Procedures**

□ Contact for Research Questions**
□ Contact for Injury Questions**
□ Contact for Research Rights Questions**
□ Participation Is Voluntary / May Discontinue**
□ More than Minimal Risk: Treatment and Compensation for Injury**
□ Number of Subjects
□ Any Costs to Subjects
□ New Findings
□ Conditions for PI Termination

	IRB Review			PI Review		
	N/A or N/R*	Yes	No	N/A or N/R*	Yes	No
The signed informed consent form is included in the participant's medical record		□	□		□	□
PHI is shared outside of the immediate research institution		□	□		□	□
If Yes Conditions for sharing PHI are clearly stated in consent form		□	□		□	□

Notes:

	IRB Review			PI Review		
a. *Amendments*	N/A or N/R*	Yes	No	N/A or N/R*	Yes	No
There have been amendments to the protocol Number: _____		☐	☐		☐	☐
Amendment #_____ Application for this amendment is on file	☐	☐	☐	☐	☐	☐
Amendment content:						
Supplementary materials were approved as part of the amendment		☐	☐		☐	☐
Amendment involved changes to the consent form		☐	☐		☐	☐
If yes, please specify:						
Approval Letter is on file Approval Date: _____		☐	☐		☐	☐
Amendment #_____ Application for this amendment is on file	☐	☐	☐	☐	☐	☐
Amendment content:						
Supplementary materials were approved as part of the amendment		☐	☐		☐	☐
Amendment involved changes to the consent form		☐	☐		☐	☐
If yes, please specify:						
Approval Letter is on file Approval Date: _____		☐	☐		☐	☐
Amendment #_____ Application for this amendment is on file	☐	☐	☐	☐	☐	☐
Amendment content:						
Supplementary materials were approved as part of the amendment		☐	☐		☐	☐
Amendment involved changes to the consent form		☐	☐		☐	☐
If yes, please specify:						
Approval Letter is on file Approval Date: _____		☐	☐		☐	☐
Amendment #_____ Application for this amendment is on file	☐	☐	☐	☐	☐	☐
Amendment content:						
Supplementary materials were approved as part of the amendment		☐	☐		☐	☐
Amendment involved changes to the consent form		☐	☐		☐	☐
If yes, please specify:						
Approval Letter is on file Approval Date: _____		☐	☐		☐	☐

	IRB Review			PI Review		
b. *Continuing Reviews*	N/A or N/R*	Yes	No	N/A or N/R*	Yes	No
There have been Continuing Reviews (CR) Number: _____	☐	☐	☐	☐	☐	☐
CR #_____ Application for this CR is on file		☐	☐		☐	☐
Approval Letter is on file Approval Date: _____		☐	☐		☐	☐
CR #_____ Application for this CR is on file		☐	☐		☐	☐
Approval Letter is on file Approval Date: _____		☐	☐		☐	☐
CR #_____ Application for this CR is on file		☐	☐		☐	☐
Approval Letter is on file Approval Date: _____		☐	☐		☐	☐
CR #_____ Application for this CR is on file		☐	☐		☐	☐
Approval Letter is on file Approval Date: _____		☐	☐		☐	☐
CR #_____ Application for this CR is on file		☐	☐		☐	☐
Approval Letter is on file Approval Date: _____		☐	☐		☐	☐
CR #_____ Application for this CR is on file		☐	☐		☐	☐
Approval Letter is on file Approval Date: _____		☐	☐		☐	☐
There was a lapse period between any protocol expiration date and the CR approval (CR #_____)	☐	☐	☐	☐	☐	☐
If Yes — Were any subjects enrolled during the lapse period?	☐	☐	☐	☐	☐	☐
If Yes — Was a protocol violation form submitted to the IRB?	☐	☐	☐	☐	☐	☐
Were any study procedures done during the lapse period?	☐	☐	☐	☐	☐	☐
If Yes — Were the procedures done during the lapse period approved by the IRB?	☐	☐	☐	☐	☐	☐
A copy of the most recent NIH or Sponsor Progress Report is on file	☐	☐	☐	☐	☐	☐
All correspondence with the IRB is on file	☐	☐	☐	☐	☐	☐

Notes:

c. *Review of Additional Sites / External IRB Approvals*		IRB Review			PI Review		
		N/A or N/R*	Yes	No	N/A or N/R*	Yes	No
The IRB is responsible for the review of additional sites	Number: _____		☐	☐		☐	☐
Name:	FWA: _____						
Location:							
Current (unexpired) approval letter is on file	Date: _____	☐	☐	☐	☐	☐	☐
Name:	FWA: _____						
Location:							
Current (unexpired) approval letter is on file	Date: _____	☐	☐	☐	☐	☐	☐
Name:	FWA: _____						
Location:							
Current (unexpired) approval letter is on file	Date: _____	☐	☐	☐	☐	☐	☐
Name:	FWA: _____						
Location:							
Current (unexpired) approval letter is on file	Date: _____	☐	☐	☐	☐	☐	☐
Name:	FWA: _____						
Location:							
Current (unexpired) approval letter is on file	Date: _____	☐	☐	☐	☐	☐	☐
There are external IRB approvals	Number: _____		☐	☐		☐	☐
Name:	FWA: _____						
Location:							
Current (unexpired) approval letter is on file	Date: _____	☐	☐	☐	☐	☐	☐
Name:	FWA: _____						
Location:							
Current (unexpired) approval letter is on file	Date: _____	☐	☐	☐	☐	☐	☐
Name:	FWA: _____						
Location:							
Current (unexpired) approval letter is on file	Date: _____	☐	☐	☐	☐	☐	☐
Name:	FWA: _____						
Location:							
Current (unexpired) approval letter is on file	Date: _____	☐	☐	☐	☐	☐	☐

	IRB Review			PI Review		
10. Adverse Events / Unexpected Problems **a. Local Events**	N/A or N/R*	Yes	No	N/A or N/R*	Yes	No
Internal Adverse Events (AEs) have occurred Number: ____ (*use additional form to report AEs if necessary*)		☐	☐		☐	☐
If Yes — Date of event: _____ ☐ Serious ☐ Unexpected ☐ Other:						
Date reported to IRB: _____						
Description:						
IRB action:						
Event was reported to DSMB, FDA, &/or sponsor (*as applicable*)	☐	☐	☐	☐	☐	☐
Date of event: _____ ☐ Serious ☐ Unexpected ☐ Other:						
Date reported to IRB: _____						
Description:						
IRB action:						
Event was reported to DSMB, FDA, &/or sponsor (*as applicable*)	☐	☐	☐	☐	☐	☐
Date of event: _____ ☐ Serious ☐ Unexpected ☐ Other:						
Date reported to IRB: _____						
Description:						
IRB action:						
Event was reported to DSMB, FDA, &/or sponsor (*as applicable*)	☐	☐	☐	☐	☐	☐
Date of event: _____ ☐ Serious ☐ Unexpected ☐ Other:						
Date reported to IRB: _____						
Description:						
IRB action:						
Event was reported to DSMB, FDA, &/or sponsor (*as applicable*)	☐	☐	☐	☐	☐	☐

Notes:

		IRB Review			PI Review		
Adverse Events / Unexpected Problems Local Events (continued)		N/A or N/R*	Yes	No	N/A or N/R*	Yes	No
Internal Unexpected Problems (UPs) have occurred Number: ____ (*use additional form to report UPs if necessary*)			☐	☐		☐	☐
If Yes	Date of event: _____ ☐ Serious ☐ Other:						
	Date reported to IRB: _____						
	Description:						
	IRB action:						
	Event was reported to DSMB, FDA, &/or sponsor (*as applicable*)	☐	☐	☐	☐	☐	☐
	Date of event: _____ ☐ Serious ☐ Other:						
	Date reported to IRB: _____						
	Description:						
	IRB action:						
	Event was reported to DSMB, FDA, &/or sponsor (*as applicable*)	☐	☐	☐	☐	☐	☐
	Date of event: _____ ☐ Serious ☐ Other:						
	Date reported to IRB: _____						
	Description:						
	IRB action:						
	Event was reported to DSMB, FDA, &/or sponsor (*as applicable*)	☐	☐	☐	☐	☐	☐
	Date of event: _____ ☐ Serious ☐ Other:						
	Date reported to IRB: _____						
	Description:						
	IRB action:						
	Event was reported to DSMB, FDA, &/or sponsor (*as applicable*)	☐	☐	☐	☐	☐	☐

Notes:

	IRB Review			PI Review		
Adverse Events / Unexpected Problems (continued) b. Off-Site Events	N/A or N/R*	Yes	No	N/A or N/R*	Yes	No
Off-Site Adverse Events (AEs) have occurred Number: ___ (*use additional form to report AEs if necessary*)		☐	☐		☐	☐
If Yes — Date of event: ___ ☐ Serious ☐ Unexpected ☐ Other:						
Date reported to IRB: ___						
Description:						
IRB action:						
Event was reported to DSMB, FDA, &/or sponsor (*as applicable*)	☐	☐	☐	☐	☐	☐
Date of event: ___ ☐ Serious ☐ Unexpected ☐ Other:						
Date reported to IRB: ___						
Description:						
IRB action:						
Event was reported to DSMB, FDA, &/or sponsor (*as applicable*)	☐	☐	☐	☐	☐	☐
Off-Site Unexpected Problems (UPs) have occurred Number: ___ (*use additional form to report UPs if necessary*)		☐	☐		☐	☐
If Yes — Date of event: ___ ☐ Serious ☐ Other:						
Date reported to IRB: ___						
Description:						
IRB action:						
Event was reported to DSMB, FDA, &/or sponsor (*as applicable*)	☐	☐	☐	☐	☐	☐
Date of event: ___ ☐ Serious ☐ Other:						
Date reported to IRB: ___						
Description:						
IRB action:						
Event was reported to DSMB, FDA, &/or sponsor (*as applicable*)	☐	☐	☐	☐	☐	☐
All AE and UP reports, IRB submissions, and IRB responses are on file		☐	☐		☐	☐

	IRB Review			PI Review		
11. Protocol Violations/Deviations/Noncompliance	N/A or N/R*	Yes	No	N/A or N/R*	Yes	No
Protocol violations have occurred Number: ____ (*use additional form to report violations if necessary*)		☐	☐		☐	☐
If Yes — Date of event: _____ ☐ Minor ☐ Significant:						
Date reported to IRB: _____						
Description:						
IRB action:						
Event was reported to DSMB, FDA, &/or sponsor (*as applicable*)	☐	☐	☐	☐	☐	☐
Date of event: _____ ☐ Minor ☐ Significant:						
Date reported to IRB: _____						
Description:						
IRB action:						
Event was reported to DSMB, FDA, &/or sponsor (*as applicable*)	☐	☐	☐	☐	☐	☐
Date of event: _____ ☐ Minor ☐ Significant						
Date reported to IRB: _____						
Description:						
IRB action:						
Event was reported to DSMB, FDA, &/or sponsor (*as applicable*)	☐	☐	☐	☐	☐	☐
For each deviation / incident of noncompliance there was adequate follow-up and resolution		☐	☐	☐	☐	☐
All deviations / incidents of noncompliance were reported to the IRB		☐	☐	☐	☐	☐
All deviations / incident reports, IRB submissions, and IRB responses are on file		☐	☐	☐	☐	☐

Notes:

		IRB Review			PI Review		
12. Drug/Device Dispensing Accountability		N/A or N/R*	Yes	No	N/A or N/R*	Yes	No
Drugs or devices are used in this study protocol			☐	☐		☐	☐
If Yes	Documentation of drug/device use for each subject is available		☐	☐		☐	☐
	Shipping/receiving is handled by: ☐ Study Site ☐ Research Pharmacy ☐ Other: _____						
	Shipping/receiving documents are on file		☐	☐		☐	☐
	A dispensing and accountability log is maintained	☐	☐	☐	☐	☐	☐
	If Yes	The log includes all necessary elements	☐	☐	☐	☐	☐	☐
		Protocol identifier	☐	☐	☐	☐	☐	☐
		Subject identifier	☐	☐	☐	☐	☐	☐
		Randomization # or Kit #	☐	☐	☐	☐	☐	☐
		Initials of person dispensing/receiving	☐	☐	☐	☐	☐	☐
		Date dispensed	☐	☐	☐	☐	☐	☐
		Amount dispensed	☐	☐	☐	☐	☐	☐
		Date returned	☐	☐	☐	☐	☐	☐
		Amount returned	☐	☐	☐	☐	☐	☐
	The drug dose is being administered and used as approved		☐	☐	☐	☐	☐	☐
	Appropriate documentation for the return/destruction of unused drugs/devices is available		☐	☐		☐	☐

Notes:

		IRB Review			PI Review	
13. Monitoring		N/A or N/R*	Yes	No	N/A or N/R*	Yes	No
This study requires a Data Safety Monitoring Plan (DSMP)		☐	☐		☐	☐
If Yes	The DSMP includes the 4 basic features	☐	☐		☐	☐
	Process to monitor research progress for patient safety	☐	☐		☐	☐
	Process of detecting and reporting adverse events (AEs)	☐	☐		☐	☐
	Process of reporting actions resulting in study suspension to the PI, Sponsor and IRB in a timely fashion	☐	☐		☐	☐
	Process for assuring data accuracy & protocol compliance	☐	☐		☐	☐
	A copy of the DSMP is on file	☐	☐		☐	☐
This study has a Data Monitoring Board (DSMB)		☐	☐		☐	☐
If Yes	Members of the DSMB are independent (not related to study conduct or interests)	☐	☐		☐	☐
	If sponsored research, at least one member of the DSMB is independent of the company	☐	☐		☐	☐
	Members of the DSMB have adequate expertise	☐	☐		☐	☐
	The DSMB has met in accordance with the IRB approved protocol	☐	☐		☐	☐
	All DSMB reports are on file	☐	☐		☐	☐
This study has had other monitoring (by sponsor, institution, QA/QI)		☐	☐		☐	☐
If Yes	Monitoring group:	☐	☐		☐	☐
	Report is on file Monitoring Date: _____	☐	☐		☐	☐
	All items that require IRB notification have been submitted	☐	☐		☐	☐
	All outstanding issues from the Monitoring Report have been addressed	☐	☐		☐	☐
	Monitoring group:	☐	☐		☐	☐
	Report is on file Monitoring Date: _____	☐	☐		☐	☐
	All items that require IRB notification have been submitted	☐	☐		☐	☐
	All outstanding issues from the Monitoring Report have been addressed	☐	☐		☐	☐
	Monitoring group:	☐	☐		☐	☐
	Report is on file Monitoring Date: _____	☐	☐		☐	☐
	All items that require IRB notification have been submitted	☐	☐		☐	☐
	All outstanding issues from the Monitoring Report have been addressed	☐	☐		☐	☐

MODEL AUDIT TOOL   Subject File

This is a model audit tool. Depending upon internal processes, information may be reviewed at different times during the preparation for or conduct of an audit. Please feel free to modify this tool so that it is appropriate for use at your institution.

General Information   Protocol Number: _____

PI Last Name: PI First Name:

	N/A or N/R	Yes	No
The PI keeps a separate study file for each participant *If no study file Is used tor each participant, completion of this form is not required*	☐	☐	☐
Record Keeping			
There is a subject log		☐	☐
Where is the subject log kept?			
There is a receipt for all subject payments	☐	☐	☐
Confidentiality is maintained in receipt documentation and payment methods		☐	☐
All consent forms are clearly organized and stored in a secure location	☐	☐	☐
Signed consents are kept separately from subject responses	☐	☐	☐

Please use this space for additional explanation/comments:

Informed Consent									N/A	Yes	No
Informed consent is required for this protocol										☐	☐
Waiver of documentation of informed consent has been approved by the IRB										☐	☐
There is a separate log to document the consent process									☐	☐	☐

Subject ID	Version (Use Valid Date)	ID on all pages of ICF		Subject Signature			PI or Study Rep signature			Witness signed (if applicable)		
	Date	Yes	No	Yes	No	Date	Yes	No	Date	Yes	No	Date
		☐	☐	☐	☐		☐	☐		☐	☐	
		☐	☐	☐	☐		☐	☐		☐	☐	
		☐	☐	☐	☐		☐	☐		☐	☐	
		☐	☐	☐	☐		☐	☐		☐	☐	
		☐	☐	☐	☐		☐	☐		☐	☐	
		☐	☐	☐	☐		☐	☐		☐	☐	
		☐	☐	☐	☐		☐	☐		☐	☐	
		☐	☐	☐	☐		☐	☐		☐	☐	
		☐	☐	☐	☐		☐	☐		☐	☐	

	N/A	Yes	No
Invalid consent forms were used (Invalid consent form includes but is not limited to: consent form without IRB approval stamp; expired consent form; incorrect study population.)		☐	☐
If Yes A protocol violation report was submitted to the IRB		☐	☐
Each subject signed the consent form in ink		☐	☐
Each participant / legally authorized representative subject dated the consent form in ink		☐	☐
The study representative signed each participant's consent form in ink		☐	☐
The study representative dated each participant's consent form in ink		☐	☐
Someone not approved by the IRB to consent subjects signed as a study representative		☐	☐
If Yes A protocol violation report was submitted to the IRB		☐	☐
Each participant received a copy of the signed and dated consent form		☐	☐
Participant's receipt of a copy of the signed and dated consent form is documented		☐	☐
A copy of the participant's signed and dated consent form is filed with Medical Records	☐	☐	☐
Informed consent was obtained and documented by parent or guardian as necessary for minors and/or cognitively impaired persons	☐	☐	☐

Please use this space for additional explanation/comments:

Minors: Informed Assent	N/A	Yes	No
Minors are enrolled		☐	☐
Invalid assent forms were used *(Invalid assent form includes but is not limited to: consent form without IRB approval stamp; expired consent form; incorrect study population.)*		☐	☐
If Yes A protocol violation report was submitted to the IRB		☐	☐
Each minor participant subject signed the assent form in ink		☐	☐
Each minor participant subject dated the assent form in ink		☐	☐
A parent/guardian signed the assent form in ink	☐	☐	☐
A parent/guardian signed a consent form in ink	☐	☐	☐
The study representative signed each minor participant's assent form	☐	☐	☐
The study representative dated each minor participant's assent form	☐	☐	☐
Someone not approved by the IRB to consent subjects signed as a study representative		☐	☐
If Yes A protocol violation report was submitted to the IRB		☐	☐
Each minor participant received a copy of the signed and dated assent form		☐	☐
The participant's receipt of a copy of the signed and dated assent form is documented		☐	☐
A copy of the minor participant's signed and dated assent form is filed with Medical Records	☐	☐	☐

Please use this space for additional explanation/comments:

Subject Selection Criteria	Yes	No
There an eligibility checklist containing inclusion/exclusion criterion	☐	☐

The participant file indicates whether the subject was included/excluded appropriately
Indicate below:

	Yes	No
Subject #1:	☐	☐
Subject #2:	☐	☐
Subject #3:	☐	☐
Subject #4:	☐	☐
Subject #5:	☐	☐
Subject #6:	☐	☐
Subject #7:	☐	☐
Subject #8:	☐	☐
Subject #9:	☐	☐
Subject #10:	☐	☐
A protocol violation was submitted to the IRB for any enrolled participants who did not meet eligibility criteria	☐	☐

The eligibility criteria checklist for each participant includes the dated signature/initials of the person obtaining the information

Subject	Yes	No	Subject	Yes	No
Subject #1:	☐	☐	Subject #6:	☐	☐
Subject #2:	☐	☐	Subject #7:	☐	☐
Subject #3:	☐	☐	Subject #8:	☐	☐
Subject #4:	☐	☐	Subject #9:	☐	☐
Subject #5:	☐	☐	Subject #10:	☐	☐

Please use this space for additional
explanation/comments:

Data Collection & Source Documents	Yes	No
There is a system in place to help staff track the progress of participants through the study procedures	☐	☐
All assessments include a subject ID number or other unique identifier	☐	☐

All subject visits / data collection is complete for the selected participants

Subject	Yes	No	Subject	Yes	No
Subject #1:	☐	☐	Subject #6:	☐	☐
Subject #2:	☐	☐	Subject #7:	☐	☐
Subject #3:	☐	☐	Subject #8:	☐	☐
Subject #4:	☐	☐	Subject #9:	☐	☐
Subject #5:	☐	☐	Subject #10:	☐	☐

If data collection is not complete, please explain:

Source documentation is available to support data entry for each subject

Subject	Yes	No	Subject	Yes	No
Subject #1:	☐	☐	Subject #6:	☐	☐
Subject #2:	☐	☐	Subject #7:	☐	☐
Subject #3:	☐	☐	Subject #8:	☐	☐
Subject #4:	☐	☐	Subject #9:	☐	☐
Subject #5:	☐	☐	Subject #10:	☐	☐
Questionnaires, surveys or other source documentation is complete				☐	☐
There adequate explanation for missing data			☐ N/A	☐	☐

If no source data or missing source documentation, please explain:

All clinical/safety tests have been reviewed by the PI or medical designee

Subject	Yes	No	Subject	Yes	No
Subject #1:	☐	☐	Subject #6:	☐	☐
Subject #2:	☐	☐	Subject #7:	☐	☐
Subject #3:	☐	☐	Subject #8:	☐	☐
Subject #4:	☐	☐	Subject #9:	☐	☐
Subject #5:	☐	☐	Subject #10:	☐	☐
If No Violations were reported to the IRB			☐ N/A	☐	☐
All clinical/safety test reviews were reviewed in a timely fashion			☐ N/A	☐	☐

Notes:

Data Collection & Source Documents (continued)

The source documentation / CRFs for each participant include dated signature/initials of the person obtaining the information for each subject

Subject	Yes	No	Subject	Yes	No
Subject #1:	☐	☐	Subject #6:	☐	☐
Subject #2:	☐	☐	Subject #7:	☐	☐
Subject #3:	☐	☐	Subject #8:	☐	☐
Subject #4:	☐	☐	Subject #9:	☐	☐
Subject #5:	☐	☐	Subject #10:	☐	☐
Changes/cross-outs in participant files are routinely initialed and dated ☐ N/A				☐	☐

Notes:

Additional Notes:

Participant File Review Eligibility *(Make copies for number of files to be reviewed)*	**Subject ID:** _____	**Subject Initials:**_____

Review of Eligibility *(complete Inclusion and exclusion fields with IRB approved protocol)*

Inclusion Criteria	Source Documentation present
☐	☐
☐	☐
☐	☐
☐	☐
☐	☐
☐	☐

Exclusion Criteria	Source Documentation present
☐	☐
☐	☐
☐	☐
☐	☐
☐	☐
☐	☐

Did the subject meet eligibility?   ☐ Yes   ☐ No

Participant File Notes:

Chapter 5
IRB Meeting Minutes Checklist

IRB MEETING MINUTES QUALITY IMPROVEMENT ASSESSMENT
Please complete one checklist for the meeting minutes for one IRB Meeting

---

IRB Panel Name

Date of Meeting

Name of Person
Completing Checklist

Date Completed

| Length of Meeting | Time Meeting Started: |
| | Time Meeting Ended: |

GENERAL MINUTES REQUIREMENTS

OHRP & FDA

1.	☐ Yes ☐ No	Do the minutes record the names of IRB members present?
2.	☐ Yes ☐ No	Do the minutes record the names of IRB members absent from the meeting?
3.	☐ Yes ☐ No ☐ N/A	Do the minutes record the names of consultants and visitors present?
4.	☐ Yes ☐ No	Does the IRB approve the minutes from the prior meeting?

AAHRPP & HURON

5.	☐ Yes ☐ No	Do the minutes record which member was chair?
6.	☐ Yes ☐ No	Do the minutes record each member's status as an unaffiliated member or affiliated member?
7.	☐ Yes ☐ No	Do the minutes record each member's status as a scientific member or non-scientific member?
8.	☐ Yes ☐ No ☐ N/A	Do the minutes record the voting status (voting or non-voting) of each member present?
9.	☐ Yes ☐ No ☐ N/A	For each alternate member, do the minutes record the name of the IRB member for whom the alternate is substituting?
10.	☐ Yes ☐ No ☐ N/A	Do the minutes record whether any members were present by teleconference and, if so, indicate them by name?
11.	☐ Yes ☐ No	Do the minutes record the total number of members present on the current IRB roster excluding alternate IRB members?
12.	☐ Yes ☐ No	Do the minutes correctly record the number of members required for a quorum? (Divide the number of members by two and select the next whole number. For example, if there are 10 IRB members on the roster, then $10/2 = 5$ and the next whole number is 6. If there are 11 IRB members on the roster, then $11/2=5.5$ and the next whole number is 6.)
13.	☐ Yes ☐ No ☐ N/A	Do the minutes record a summary/list of each business item (e.g., educational items, announcements, etc.) that was discussed?

14.	☐ Yes ☐ No	Do the minutes record acknowledgment of expedited actions (including approvals, continuing reviews, and amendments) carried out since the last meeting?
		If not, how are these approvals communicated to IRB members?
15.	☐ Yes ☐ No	Do the minutes record the chair's conflict of interest (COI) reminder?
16.	☐ Yes ☐ No ☐ N/A	For protocols undergoing continuing review by full committee, does the convened IRB (with quorum) review, deliberate, and vote for each study?
17.	☐ Yes ☐ No ☐ N/A	Do the minutes document IRB review of adverse events and unanticipated problems?
18.	☐ Yes ☐ No ☐ N/A	Do the minutes include IRB review of protocol violations or deviations?

INSTITUTIONAL REQUIREMENTS
(Please include policies specific to your institution that should be included in your minutes)

19.	☐ Yes ☐ No	
20.	☐ Yes ☐ No	
21.	☐ Yes ☐ No	

REQUIREMENTS FOR EACH PROTOCOL OR REPORT REVIEWED

OHRP & FDA

22.	☐ Yes ☐ No ☐ N/A	For each protocol reviewed by the IRB, do the minutes include written documentation of any discussion of controverted issues and their resolution?
23.	☐ Yes ☐ No ☐ N/A	For protocols in which the IRB waived the requirement of informed consent, was the justification for the waiver documented in the minutes in accordance with 45 CFR 46.116(d)?
24.	☐ Yes ☐ No ☐ N/A	For research involving pregnant women and/or fetuses, do the minutes document IRB findings required under Subpart B of 45 CFR 46?
25.	☐ Yes ☐ No ☐ N/A	For research involving prisoners, does the composition of the IRB include a prisoner or a prisoner representative with appropriate background and experience?
26.	☐ Yes ☐ No ☐ N/A	For research involving prisoners, do the minutes document IRB findings as required under 45 CFR 46.305(a)?
27.	☐ Yes ☐ No ☐ N/A	For research involving children, do the minutes document IRB findings in accordance with Subpart D of 45 CFR 46?
28.	☐ Yes ☐ No ☐ N/A	Do the minutes document consideration of additional safeguards for vulnerable subjects when appropriate?
29.	☐ Yes ☐ No	Do the minutes document that a quorum was present for all IRB actions requiring a vote?
30.	☐ Yes ☐ No	Do the minutes document that at least a majority of the IRB members present voted on all actions requiring a vote?
31.	☐ Yes ☐ No	Do the minutes document that all IRB actions included at least one scientist in the review and vote?

32.	☐ Yes ☐ No	Do the minutes document that all IRB actions included at least one non-scientist in the review and vote?
33.	☐ Yes ☐ No	Do the minutes document that all IRB actions included at least one non-institutional member in the review and vote?
		If not, how frequently has the absence of this member occurred in the past three months?
34.	☐ Yes ☐ No	Do the minutes of the IRB meetings include sufficient detail to show the vote on the IRB's actions including the number of members voting for, against, and abstaining?
35.	☐ Yes ☐ No ☐ N/A	Do the minutes record the name of IRB members who abstained from a vote and provide the reason for abstention?
36.	☐ Yes ☐ No ☐ N/A	Do the minutes record the name of IRB members who recused themselves from the discussion and vote due to a conflict of interest?
		If yes, was the reason for the conflict documented in the minutes?
37.	☐ Yes ☐ No ☐ N/A	When specific minor modifications are required to approve a study, do the IRB minutes state who (e.g., chair, reviewers, full committee) will review and confirm that the investigator has completed the modifications requested by the IRB?

AAHRPP & HURON

38.	☐ Yes ☐ No	Do the minutes record a protocol number? (May not be applicable for Reportable New Information with no specific protocol involved.)
39.	☐ Yes ☐ No	Do the minutes record a study title? (May not be applicable for Reportable New Information with no specific protocol involved.)
40.	☐ Yes ☐ No	Do the minutes record the principal investigator's name? (May not be applicable for Reportable New Information with no specific protocol involved.)
41.	☐ Yes ☐ No	Do the minutes record a type of review as initial review, continuing review, review of modifications to previously approved research, or reportable new information?
42.	☐ Yes ☐ No ☐ N/A	If the minutes record a consultant report, does it summarize the key information provided the consultant. ("N/A" if there were no consultant reports.)
43.	☐ Yes ☐ No	Do the minutes record a motion as one of the following: Approved, Requires Modifications, Deferred, or Disapproved. (May not be applicable for Reportable New Information.)
44.	☐ Yes ☐ No ☐ N/A	For initial or continuing review, do the minutes record the period of approval for the motion?
45.	☐ Yes ☐ No	Do the minutes record the number of members for, against, abstaining, absent, or recused for each vote?
46.	☐ Yes ☐ No ☐ N/A	Do the minutes list the names of IRB members who were absent or recused for each vote?
47.	☐ Yes ☐ No ☐ N/A	Do the minutes document the level of risk determined by the convened IRB as either minimal risk or greater than minimal risk?

48.	☐ Yes ☐ No ☐ N/A	If the research involves waiver or alteration of consent, waiver of written documentation of consent, inclusion of children, pregnant women, neonates, fetuses, prisoners, do the minutes either say "See IRB Records" or include documentation that the criteria were met? ("N/A" if no research requiring documented findings was reviewed.)
49.	☐ Yes ☐ No ☐ N/A	Do minutes justify any deletion or substantive modification of information concerning risks or alternative procedures contained in the DHHS-approved sample consent document? ("N/A" if a DHHS-approved sample consent form was not reviewed.)
50.	☐ Yes ☐ No ☐ N/A	Do the minutes document the determination of need for an Investigational New Drug Application (IND)?
51.	☐ Yes ☐ No ☐ N/A	Do minutes document the rationale for a significant/non-significant device determination? ("N/A" if abbreviated IDE devices were not reviewed.)
52.	☐ Yes ☐ No ☐ N/A	Do minutes document modifications required to secure approval? ("N/A" if there were no modifications required to secure approval.)
53.	☐ Yes ☐ No ☐ N/A	When minutes document modifications required to secure approval is a reason (basis) for each modification included? ("N/A" if there were no modifications required to secure approval.)
54.	☐ Yes ☐ No ☐ N/A	If a protocol was deferred or disapproved, do the minutes document the reasons? ("N/A" if there were no deferred or disapproved protocols.)
55.	☐ Yes ☐ No ☐ N/A	If a protocol was deferred, do the minutes document recommended changes? ("N/A" if there were no deferred or disapproved protocols.)
56.	☐ Yes ☐ No ☐ N/A	If both a regular IRB member and the alternate IRB member are present at the meeting, do the minutes indicate which voted and record the vote of just one? ("N/A" if both a regular IRB member and the alternate IRB member were not present at the meeting.)
57.	☐ Yes ☐ No	Is the sum total of the number of members for, against, abstaining, absent, or recused constant among votes and equal to the number of people listed in the meeting attendance roster?
58.	☐ Yes ☐ No ☐ N/A	For each Reportable New Information (RNI) reviewed, do the minutes describe the new information? ("N/A" if no RNIs were reviewed
59.	☐ Yes ☐ No ☐ N/A	For each Reportable New Information (RNI) reviewed, do the minutes describe whether the new information was serious or continuing noncompliance, an unanticipated problem involving risks to subjects or others, or a suspension or termination of IRB approval? ("N/A" if no RNIs were reviewed.)
60.	☐ Yes ☐ No ☐ N/A	For each Reportable New Information (RNI) reviewed, do the minutes describe whether the IRB members considered termination of IRB approval? ("N/A" if no RNIs were reviewed.)
61.	☐ Yes ☐ No ☐ N/A	For each Reportable New Information (RNI) reviewed, do the minutes document the required action(s) of the Investigator and/or IRB? ("N/A" if no RNIs were reviewed.)
62.	☐ Yes ☐ No ☐ N/A	For each Reportable New Information (RNI) reviewed, do the minutes document the motion? ("N/A" if no RNIs were reviewed.)
63.	☐ Yes ☐ No ☐ N/A	If the minutes record controverted issues, is there a "Controverted Issue / Resolution" table? ("N/A" if there were no controverted issues.)
64.	☐ Yes ☐ No ☐ N/A	If the "Controverted Issue / Resolution" table was used, does it summarize the controverted issue? ("N/A" if there were no controverted issues.)

| 65. | ☐ Yes ☐ No ☐ N/A | If the "Controverted Issue / Resolution" table was used, does it include a resolution or a statement that there was no resolution? ("N/A" if there were no controverted issues.) |
| 66. | ☐ Yes ☐ No ☐ N/A | If appropriate, do the minutes record research data security issues and resolutions? |

OPTIONAL QUESTIONS *(Questions were taken from the OHRP QA Self-Assessment Tool)*

Estimated amount of time for full committee
protocols/meeting

Estimated amount of time for modifications
requiring full committee review/meeting

Estimated amount of time for review of adverse
reactions / unanticipated events reported /
meeting

Estimated amount of time for continuing review
protocols requiring full committee review/meeting

IRB Membership Composition Audit Checklist

	Check box if statement is fulfilled
☐	At least five members, not including alternate IRB members.
☐	At least one member whose primary concerns are in scientific areas.
☐	At least one member whose primary concerns are in non-scientific areas.
☐	At least one member who is not otherwise affiliated with the institution and who is not part of the immediate family of a person who is affiliated with the institution.
☐	Sufficient alternate IRB members with appropriate qualifications appointed and willing to serve.
☐	An appointed IRB chair.
☐	Be of varying backgrounds including race, gender, and culture.
☐	Be of varying backgrounds to promote and complete an adequate review of research activities commonly conducted by the institution.
☐	Be sufficiently qualified through the experience and expertise of its members (professional competence), and the diversity of its members and sensitivity to such issues as community attitudes, to promote respect for its advice and counsel in safeguarding the rights and welfare of human subjects.
☐	Be able to ascertain the acceptability of proposed research in terms of institutional commitments (including policies and resources) and regulations, applicable law, and standards of professional conduct and practice.
☐	If an IRB regularly reviews research that involves a category of subjects that is vulnerable to coercion or undue influence, such as children, prisoners, individuals with impaired decision-making capacity, or economically or educationally disadvantaged persons, consideration shall be given to the inclusion of one or more individuals who are knowledgeable about and experienced in working with these categories of subjects.
☐	No IRB may have a member participate in the IRB's initial or continuing review of any project in which the member has a conflicting interest, except to provide information requested by the IRB.
☐	A majority of the Board (exclusive of *Prisoner* members) has no association with the prison(s) involved, apart from their membership on the Board.
☐	At least one voting member of the Board is a *Prisoner*, or a *Prisoner* representative with appropriate background and experience to serve in that capacity, including a working knowledge of the population to be recruited, a reasonable familiarity with the operations of the prison or confinement facility, and any other legally imposed restrictive conditions involved in the research. (The prisoner representative may be an alternate member who becomes a voting member when needed.)

Other items to consider:

- The roster of IRB members must include name, earned degrees, representative capacity, indications of experience, and any employment or other relationship between each member and the institution.
- Any IRB member who has a conflict of interest with regard to a specific protocol may provide information to the IRB if asked but may not be part of the IRB discussion or vote.
- An IRB may use consultants for topic areas of review where the expertise on the IRB is not sufficient; the consultant serves as a non-voting member.
- No protocol can be approved in the absence of a non-scientific member or an alternate for the non-scientific member; meeting is not appropriately constituted convened IRB meeting. Discussion may be held.

- If the protocol involves a specific category of vulnerable populations, a voting IRB member who has relevant research expertise must be present.
- If the research involves prisoners, at least one member of the IRB must be a prisoner or prisoner representative with appropriate background and experience, and a majority of the IRB cannot have any association with the prisons involved in the research.

Appendix C
Investigator Toolkit

Note-to-File Template

PROTOCOL #:	*[insert protocol #]*
TITLE:	*[insert subject title]*
Re:	*[insert topic of note / event and study subject number if needed]*
Date:	*[insert date]*

Description

[insert description]

Action(s) Taken

[insert any action taken and any recommendations]

Signature:

Role in Study: **Date:**

Regulatory Binder Tabs Template
Regulatory Binder Instructions

INSTRUCTIONS

This regulatory binder is available to help study sites achieve and maintain regulatory compliance and adhere to high standards of practice in the conduct of research involving human subjects.

Each section outlines the regulatory documentation requirements, general guidance for organization and record keeping, and, when applicable, references to federal regulations and Good Clinical Practice guidelines.

GENERAL GUIDANCE FOR USING THE REGULATORY BINDER

- Tailor the binder to meet the needs of your specific protocol:
  - □ This regulatory binder is a template. Include only sections pertinent to your protocol. Omit unused sections and add sections as needed. See "Applicable sections" below for more information.
  - □ Organize and order the sections to facilitate easy use and reference, e.g., file most used and referenced sections in the front of the binder.
  - □ Add additional tabs and/or documents to each section as needed.
- Keep the regulatory binder current and up to date.
- Identify an individual(s) responsible for maintaining the binder. Ensure that this person is on file with the IRB as an additional person to contact to ensure that all IRB correspondence and documents are received/filed in a timely manner.
- Store binder in a safe and secure location but accessible to study staff at all times.
- Participant-specific documentation and information, e.g., signed consent forms, test results, and completed case report forms, should be maintained separately in participant-specific binder/file.

WHAT SECTIONS APPLY TO YOUR RESEARCH PROTOCOL

Depending on the nature of the research, some tabs may or may not be required. Use the list below to ensure that the applicable sections are maintained.

Regulatory Binder Essentials

- Protocol
- CVs, Licensure, Trainings
- IRB Documentation
- Study Logs
- Consent Forms
- Data Collection

If FDA-regulated Human Research (e.g. IND, IDE) include the below tabs in addition to the essentials listed above:

- Investigator Brochure, Pack Insert, or Device Manual
- Drug/Device-related information
- FDA Documentation
- Sponsor Correspondence/Documentation
- Logs
  - Screening/Enrollment
  - AE/SAE/Protocol Deviations
  - Monitoring / Site Visits
  - Delegation of Responsibility
  - Investigational Product Dispensation / Accountability

If the Human Research involves labs, include the below tabs in addition to the essentials listed above:

- CLIA/CAP certifications
- Current/past lab normal ranges

Other tabs (if applicable):

- NIH
- External IRB Documentation
- Ethics Committee / Community Advisory Board Documentation
- Scientific Review
- Data Safety Monitoring Board
- Data Protection

Protocol

REQUIREMENTS

☐ Original Protocol and all amended versions

☐ All versions should contain a version date and/or number

☐ If applicable, include copy of fully executed protocol signature page for original protocol with signed principal investigator (PI) signature page

GUIDANCE

✓ If documents are maintained electronically, write a note-to-file indicating the location and who maintains them (include copy of note-to-file here).

FEDERAL REGULATIONS / GOOD CLINICAL PRACTICE

GCP: 8.2.2; 8.3.2

CVs

REQUIREMENTS

☐ CVs for all study staff

GUIDANCE

✓ CVs should be signed, dated, and updated every 2 years to verify that the information is accurate and current.

✓ If CVs are filed collectively for the department, write a signed and dated note-to-file indicating the location (include copy of note-to-file here).

✓ If CVs are maintained electronically, write a note-to-file indicating the location and who maintains them (include copy of note-to-file here).

✓ For NIH funded studies, investigators can use their NIH Bio Sketch.

FEDERAL REGULATIONS / GOOD CLINICAL PRACTICE

GCP: 4.1.1; 8.2.10; 8.3.5

Licensure

REQUIREMENTS

☐ Valid licenses/certification for all professional study staff (e.g., medical or nursing license)

☐ Current professional certification, as indicated

GUIDANCE

✓ If documents are maintained electronically, write a note-to-file indicating the location and who maintains them (include copy of note-to-file here).

✓ In MA, medical and nursing licenses must be renewed every 2 years. Licensure renewal dates coincide with birth dates. It is important to monitor licensure expiration dates so that those nearing expiration can be promptly replaced.

✓ Professional certification information should be included in individual CVs. The frequency with which certification must be renewed varies widely, depending on the requirements of the certifying body.

FEDERAL REGULATIONS / GOOD CLINICAL PRACTICE

GCP: 4.1.1, 8.2.10

Training

REQUIREMENTS

☐ Human research training

☐ Additional training certification of study staff, e.g., phlebotomy, vital signs, etc.)

☐ Sponsor training (e.g., EDC trainings, study initiation visits, use of device, GCP)

☐ Institution specific training

GUIDANCE

✓ If documents are maintained electronically, write a note-to-file indicating the location and who maintains them (include copy of note-to-file here).

FEDERAL REGULATIONS / GOOD CLINICAL PRACTICE

GCP: 4.1.1

IRB Documentation

REQUIREMENTS

☐ Copies of signed and dated submissions:
- Initial Application for Human Research
- Continuing Review(s)
- Modifications/Amendments
- Reportable New Information
- Adverse Events
- Protocol Violations
- Unanticipated Problems

☐ Original Approval letters and/or notification of IRB decisions

☐ Copy of investigator response to IRB notification (if applicable)

☐ Approved/validated recruitment materials

☐ Approved/validated additional study information distributed to participants

☐ Any foreign language materials (if applicable)

☐ Print out of Institution's FWA Information from OHRP website

☐ IRB Membership Roster*

☐ Any additional correspondence related to the study (e.g. e-mails)

   * Required for FDA-regulated protocols

GUIDANCE

✓ Submissions should be signed and dated as applicable. If your institution uses an electronic system for submitting and storing IRB documents, ensure that the electronic file contains all required documents and write a note-to-file indicating the location (include copy of note-to-file here).

✓ File documents in reverse chronological order.

✓ Request a copy of missing documentation from your institutional representative.

FEDERAL REGULATIONS / GOOD CLINICAL PRACTICE
GCP: 8.2.7, 8.2.9, 8.3.2-8.3.4

Study Logs
CHECK ALL THAT ARE INCLUDED:

☐ Screening Log

☐ Enrollment Log

☐ Staff Signature Log

☐ Delegation of Authority/Responsibility Log

☐ Study Monitoring / Site Visit Log*

☐ Adverse Event Tracking Log

☐ Protocol Deviation/Exception Tracking Log

☐ Specimen Log

☐ Training Log

Required for FDA-regulated protocols

GUIDANCE

✓ Update logs in a timely manner. To ensure accuracy, logs should be updated as soon as possible after a recordable event occurs, preferable on the same day.

✓ If documents are maintained electronically, write a note-to-file indicating the location and who maintains them (include copy of note-to-file here).

FEDERAL REGULATIONS / GOOD CLINICAL PRACTICE
GCP: 8.3.20-8.3.25

Consent Forms

REQUIREMENTS

☐ Original copies of all IRB approved versions (evident by the IRB approval/validation stamp) with version dates or numbers

☐ Copies of foreign language consent materials, if applicable

GUIDANCE

✓ If documents are maintained electronically, write a note-to-file indicating the location and who maintains them (include copy of note-to-file here).

FEDERAL REGULATIONS / GOOD CLINICAL PRACTICE

HHS: 45 CFR 46

FDA: 21 CFR 50; 21 CFR 56

GCP: 8.2.3; 8.2.7; 8.3.2; 8.3.12

Data Collection

REQUIREMENTS

☐ Blank set of case report forms (CRFs), data collection sheets, and/or study questionnaires

GUIDANCE

✓ If documents are maintained electronically, write a note-to-file indicating the location and who maintains them (include copy of note-to-file here).

✓ The difference between data collection sheets and case report forms is that data collection sheets typically act as source documentation. That is, during study visits, information is written directly onto the worksheets. An industry sponsor usually provides CRFs; all protocol-required information is transferred to CRFs from data collection sheets. Some studies do not use CRFs. All studies should use some type of data collection sheet.

FEDERAL REGULATIONS / GOOD CLINICAL PRACTICE
FDA: 21 CFR 312.53; 312.62
GCP: 8.3.14; 8.3.15; 4.9.3

Investigator Brochure / Pack Insert / Device Manual
REQUIREMENTS

☐ Most recent version of investigator brochure or product information,
   e.g., package insert or sample label (for investigational drugs)
☐ Device Manual or Report of Prior Investigations, ROPI (for investigational devices)

GUIDANCE

✓ Send updated versions to the IRB.
✓ If the investigational product is marketed and its pharmacology is
   widely understood, a basic product information brochure or package
   insert may be an appropriate alternative.
✓ If documents are maintained electronically, write a note-to-file indicating the location and who maintains them (include copy of note-
   to-file here).

FEDERAL REGULATIONS / GOOD CLINICAL PRACTICE
FDA: 21 CFR 312.55
GCP: 8.2.1; 8.3.1

Drug/Device

REQUIREMENTS

☐ Drug/Device Accountability Log

☐ Drug/Device Dispensing Log

☐ Drug/Device Shipment and Receipt Records

GUIDANCE

✓ The PI is responsible for the following with respect to investigational drugs/devices:

- Maintain records of investigational product delivery to the study site. Include dates, quantities received, batch/serial numbers, and expiration dates.

- Maintain an inventory of the investigational product at any site. Inventory control records should be updated, signed, and dated by the PI in a timely manner.

- Record/track use of the investigational product by each participant. Documentation should verify that dosing / device use was in accordance with the approved protocol. Maintain an accountability log that records when the participant(s) received the drugs/device and the specific dosage/device the participant(s) received.

- Return/dispose of unused investigational product as specified by the sponsor. Maintain documentation of return/disposal.

- Store the investigational product. The storage area should be locked/secure with access limited to approved study staff only. Drugs/devices should not be stored with standard clinical inventory.

✓ If applicable, write a signed and dated note-to-file indicating where documentation is kept (e.g. Research Pharmacy). Include the note-to-file here.

✓ If documents are maintained electronically, write a note-to-file indicating the location and who maintains them (include copy of note-to-file behind tab).

✓ If drug/device shipment, receipt, and accountability are managed by the research pharmacy, include note-to-file here.

FEDERAL REGULATIONS / GOOD CLINICAL PRACTICE
FDA: 21 CFR 312.57; 312.62; 812.140

FDA Documentation

REQUIREMENTS

Clinical Investigator:

☐ Copy of all versions of the Form FDA 1572 (for investigational drugs)
☐ Copy of all versions of Investigator Agreement (for investigational devices)
☐ Copy of all Safety Reports submitted to the FDA

Financial Disclosure:

☐ Signed and dated copy of all Form FDA 3455 (Disclosure: Financial Interests and arrangements of Clinical Investigators)

Sponsor-Investigator:

☐ Copy of all Form FDA 1571 submitted to the FDA (for investigational drugs only), Initial IND/IDE or Application
☐ Amendments/Supplements to the application
☐ Safety Reports
☐ Annual Progress Reports
☐ Form 3674, certification of registration to ClinicalTrials.gov

GUIDANCE

✓ The Form FDA 1571 should be used as the cover sheet for all correspondence sent to the FDA.
✓ Instructions for completing The Form FDA 1572 can be found at: https://www.fda.gov/media/77596/download.
✓ Update the 1572 each time there is a change to any of the information originally provided. Notify the Sponsor of updates.
✓ If documents are maintained electronically, write a note-to-file indicating the location and who maintains them (include copy of note-to-file here).

FEDERAL REGULATIONS / GOOD CLINICAL PRACTICE
FDA: 21 CFR 54; 312.30; 312.32; 312.33; 812.150(b)(1); 812.150(b)(5); 812.35; 812.43(c)

Sponsor

REQUIREMENTS

□ All correspondence to and from the sponsor (e.g. letters, meeting notes, and notes of telephone calls)

□ Signed Agreements, including Financial Agreements

□ Insurance Statement (when required)

GUIDANCE

✓ If documents are maintained electronically, write a note-to-file indicating the location and who maintains them (include copy of note-to-file here).

Laboratory

REQUIREMENTS

☐ Lab certification (e.g. CLIA, CAP) and updates
☐ Normal lab/reference values and updates
☐ Lab Director's CV
☐ Handling Instructions (if not specified in Investigator's Brochure, Device Manual, or Package Insert)

GUIDANCE

✓ Keep updated documents to exhibit the competency of all lab facilities being utilized, and to support the reliability of test results.
✓ If documents are filed separately or maintained electronically, write a note-to-file indicating the location and who maintains them (include copy of note-to-file here).
✓ Research labs typically do not have lab certifications (e.g., CLIA, CAP) and may not have "normal" lab values. If research labs are used, ensure that the lab director's CV and research lab references values are on file.

FEDERAL REGULATIONS / GOOD CLINICAL PRACTICE
GCP: 8.2.11; 8.2.12; 8.2.14; 8.3.6; 8.3.7

NIH

REQUIREMENTS

☐ Copy of the NIH grant application and progress reports

GUIDANCE

✓ Submit a copy of the most recent progress report as specified by your IRB.

✓ Any additional study correspondence (e.g., e-mails) with the NIH and Collaborators.

✓ If documents are maintained electronically, write a note-to-file indicating the location and who maintains them (include copy of note-to-file here).

External IRB Documentation

Instructions: Use this binder tab to maintain documentation from external, US-based, institutions (e.g., Veteran's Affairs, additional site conducting concurrent IRB review).

REQUIREMENTS

• External IRB documentation, including IRB submissions, IRB notifications, and significant correspondence between the IRB and investigator.
• Documentation of an institution's agreement to rely on another for IRB review, e.g., protocol-specific IRB Authorization Agreement, acknowledgement letter demonstrating cede review.

DOCUMENTATION TIPS

• If documentation is maintained electronically, write a note-to-file indicating the location and who maintains them (include copy of note-to-file here).
• If helpful, maintain links to applicable local, regional, and/or national regulation/guidance on file.
• To reduce the administrative burden of concurrent IRB review, consider an IRB Authorization Agreement whereby one institution relies on another for IRB review.
• Investigators must follow their institution's policies and procedures. Contact your institution for additional guidance.

Ethics Committee / Community Advisory Board

Instructions: Use this binder tab when conducting international research to maintain local host-country Ethics Committee (EC) and/ or Community Advisory Board (CAB) documentation, including applicable local, regional, and/or national reviewing bodies in host country site(s).

REQUIREMENTS

- EC or CAB documentation, including complete submissions, notifications, and significant correspondence.

DOCUMENTATION TIPS

- It is insufficient for a US-based institution to approve non-exempt human research conducted abroad. Local ethical review is required.
- For Health and Human Service-funded protocols:
  - The review is recommended by the EC of an engaged organization or that of another organization in the same geographic area.
  - The local EC should be registered with the Office for Human Research Protections and have a federal wide assurance.
- For non-Health and Human Service-funded protocols:
  - Review is recommended by a local EC or CAB.
- When documentation is maintained locally in the host country and/or electronically, use a note-to-file to document their location and who is responsible.
- If helpful, maintain links to applicable local, regional, and/or national regulation/guidance on file.

Scientific Review

REQUIREMENTS

☐ Copy of materials submitted for scientific review

☐ Original, signed notification letters (when applicable)

GUIDANCE

✓ If documents are maintained electronically, write a note-to-file indicating the location and who maintains them (include copy of note-to-file here).

Data Safety Monitoring Board

REQUIREMENTS

☐ Copy of all documentation for data safety monitoring plan as out-lined in the IRB approved protocol
☐ Copy of all DSMB reports
☐ Copy of all audit reports (internal and external)

GUIDANCE

✓ If your study has a DSMB, submit a copy of the most recent DSMB report to the IRB at the time of continuing review.
✓ Any additional correspondence (e.g. e-mails, letters, meeting min-utes) with the DSMB and its members.
✓ If documents are maintained electronically, write a note-to-file indi-cating the location and who maintains them (include copy of note-to-file here).

FEDERAL REGULATIONS / GOOD CLINICAL PRACTICE
GCP: 8.3.10; 5.19.3

Data Protection

RECOMMENDED CONTENTS:

- ☐ Data Collection/Use Plan (if not in the IRB approved protocol)
- ☐ Data Storage Plan (if not in the IRB approved protocol)
- ☐ Data Transfer/Sharing Plan (if not in the IRB approved protocol)
- ☐ Data Management Plan (if not in the IRB approved protocol)
  - Protection and security of research data
  - Risk Management, which includes data breach and response
- ☐ Data Retention/Return and/or Destruction Plan
- ☐ Data Use Agreements or other agreements/contracts pertaining to data sharing with external collaborators, vendors, and/or third-party business associates (signed and dated by all parties)
- ☐ Documentation of Authorization to use protected health information for research purposes (in informed consent form or stand-alone authorization)
- ☐ Waiver of HIPAA Authorization (if applicable)

GUIDANCE

- ✓ If documents are maintained electronically, write a note-to-file indicating the location and who maintains them (include copy of note-to-file here).
- ✓ Investigators must follow their institution's policies and procedures. Refer to the following links for institution-specific research data security policies or contact your institution for additional guidance.

FEDERAL AND STATE REGULATIONS

OCR: HIPAA Privacy Rule and Security Rule (as amended):
HHS: 45 CFR 160, 162 and 164 (Subparts A and C)
FDA: FDA: 21 CFR, Part 11

Investigator Self-Assessment

HUMAN RESEARCH (Non-Clinical Trials)	
Principal Investigator	
Protocol # / Study Title	/
Name of Person Completing Checklist	
Date Completed	

The purpose of this checklist is to allow investigators to conduct a quality improvement self-assessment and/or for QA/QI staff to conduct quality improvement assessments of investigators. This section is designed for research studies that are NOT considered clinical trials. Please complete this section if the research study you are conducting is considered Social, Behavioral, or Education research.

1. Regulatory Documentation for Each Study

☐ Yes ☐ No ☐ N/A	Grant	
☐ Yes ☐ No ☐ N/A	Sponsor's Agreement, Contract	
☐ Yes ☐ No ☐ N/A	Annual progress reports for grant Total Number:	
☐ Yes ☐ No ☐ N/A	Most recent version of the IRB approved protocol	
☐ Yes ☐ No ☐ N/A	Previous versions of the IRB approved protocol Total Number:	
☐ Yes ☐ No ☐ N/A	Most recent version of the IRB approved recruitment materials	
☐ Yes ☐ No ☐ N/A	Previous versions of the IRB approved recruitment materials Total Number:	
☐ Yes ☐ No ☐ N/A	Most recent version of the IRB approved consent document(s)	
☐ Yes ☐ No ☐ N/A	Previous versions of the IRB approved consent document(s) Total Number:	
☐ Yes ☐ No ☐ N/A	Most recent version of the IRB approved parental permission/assent document(s)	
☐ Yes ☐ No ☐ N/A	Previous versions of the IRB approved parental permission/assent document(s) Total Number:	
☐ Yes ☐ No ☐ N/A	Most recent version of the IRB approved study tools, e.g., survey/questionnaire	

☐ Yes ☐ No ☐ N/A		Previous versions of the IRB approved study tools, e.g., survey/questionnaire Total Number:
☐ Yes ☐ No ☐ N/A		Correspondence with the IRB on file: (look for signature and date when needed for submission)
☐ Yes ☐ No ☐ N/A		Initial IRB application
☐ Yes ☐ No ☐ N/A		Continuing review(s). Total Number:
☐ Yes ☐ No ☐ N/A		Modification Request(s). Total Number:
☐ Yes ☐ No ☐ N/A		Reportable New Information form(s). Total Number:
☐ Yes ☐ No ☐ N/A		Notifications of IRB disapproval, deferral, modifications required to secure approval
☐ Yes ☐ No ☐ N/A		Responses to IRB actions
☐ Yes ☐ No ☐ N/A		IRB suspensions or terminations
☐ Yes ☐ No ☐ N/A		Copies of e-mail correspondence with the IRB
☐ Yes ☐ No ☐ N/A		Other communications with the IRB
☐ Yes ☐ No ☐ N/A		Records of investigator and study staff human research training
☐ Yes ☐ No ☐ N/A		Training certificates are valid (completed within the past 3 years or other applicable period, per institutional policy)
☐ Yes ☐ No ☐ N/A		CVs or other relevant documents (biosketch/resume) evidencing qualifications of PI, co-investigators, and all study personnel
☐ Yes ☐ No ☐ N/A		CVs / other relevant information have been updated within the past two years or other applicable period, per institutional policy)
☐ Yes ☐ No ☐ N/A		CVs / other relevant information are signed and dated
☐ Yes ☐ No ☐ N/A		Signed agreements/contracts between parties (e.g., MOA, DUA, LDT)
☐ Yes ☐ No ☐ N/A		Correspondences to and from the funding agency
☐ Yes ☐ No ☐ N/A		IRB roster
☐ Yes ☐ No ☐ N/A		Documentation of IRB's Federalwide Assurance (FWA) Number

2. Document Retention

☐ Yes ☐ No ☐ N/A	Regulatory documentation (e.g., contents of the Regulatory Binder) are retained for at least XXXXX years after closing out the Human Research	
☐ Yes ☐ No ☐ N/A	Records for sponsored research are retained until the sponsor authorized destruction of the records. Instructions or date of authorized destruction:	

3. Subject Recruitment Procedures

☐ Yes ☐ No ☐ N/A	Are the IRB-approved recruitment methods being followed?
☐ Yes ☐ No ☐ N/A	Have all recruitment materials (e.g., advertisements and telephone scripts) been approved by the IRB? Note: ALL recruitment materials must be approved prior to use and must be reapproved at the time of continuing review.

4. Data and Safety Monitoring

☐ Yes ☐ No ☐ N/A	Is there a Data Safety Monitoring Plan (DSMP) for this study?
☐ Yes ☐ No ☐ N/A	Has the DSMP been followed per the IRB approved protocol?
☐ Yes ☐ No ☐ N/A	Is there a Data and Safety Monitoring Board (DSMB) for this study?
☐ Yes ☐ No ☐ N/A	Have all DSMB reports been submitted to the IRB? Total Number:

CLINICAL TRIALS

Principal Investigator	
Protocol # / Study Title	/
Name of Person Completing Checklist	
Date Completed	

The purpose of this checklist is to allow investigators to conduct a quality improvement self-assessment and/or for QA/QI staff to conduct quality improvement assessments of investigators. This section is designed for Clinical Trials.[1] The reviewer should identify and complete the applicable sections for each unique study.

1. Regulatory Documentation[2]

☐ Yes   ☐ No   ☐ N/A   Grant

☐ Yes   ☐ No   ☐ N/A   Sponsor's Agreement, Contract

☐ Yes   ☐ No   ☐ N/A   Annual progress reports for grant
Total Number:

☐ Yes   ☐ No   ☐ N/A   Most recent version of the IRB approved protocol

☐ Yes   ☐ No   ☐ N/A   Previous versions of the IRB approved protocol
Total Number:

☐ Yes   ☐ No   ☐ N/A   Most recent version of the IRB approved recruitment materials

☐ Yes   ☐ No   ☐ N/A   Previous versions of the IRB approved recruitment materials
Total Number:

☐ Yes   ☐ No   ☐ N/A   Most recent version of the IRB approved consent document(s)

☐ Yes   ☐ No   ☐ N/A   Previous versions of the IRB approved consent document(s)
Total Number:

☐ Yes   ☐ No   ☐ N/A   Most recent version of the IRB approved parental permission/assent document(s)

☐ Yes   ☐ No   ☐ N/A   Previous versions of the IRB approved parental permission/assent document(s)
Total Number:

1. FDA defines Clinical Investigation as, "Clinical investigation means any experiment that involves a test article and one or more human subjects and that either is subject to requirements for prior submission to the Food and Drug Administration under section 505(i) or 520(g) of the act, or is not subject to requirements for prior submission to the Food and Drug Administration under these sections of the act, but the results of which are intended to be submitted later to, or held for inspection by, the Food and Drug Administration as part of an application for a research or marketing permit. The term does not include experiments that are subject to the provisions of part 58 of this chapter, regarding nonclinical laboratory studies." (http://www.accessdata.fda.gov/scripts/cdrh/cfdocs/cfcfr/CFRSearch.cfm?fr=50.3). NIH defines Clinical Trial as, "A research study in which one or more human subjects are prospectively assigned to one or more interventions (which may include placebo or other control) to evaluate the effects of those interventions on health-related biomedical or behavioral outcomes" (http://grants.nih.gov/grants/guide/notice-files/NOT-OD-15-015.html).

2. Copies of correspondences may be retained in hardcopy or electronic format (e.g., shared folder space).

☐ Yes	☐ No	☐ N/A	Most recent version of IRB approved information, e.g., brochure, information sheet, results letter, etc.
☐ Yes	☐ No	☐ N/A	Previous versions of IRB approved information, e.g., brochure, information sheet, results letter, etc. Total Number:
☐ Yes	☐ No	☐ N/A	Most recent version of the IRB approved study tools, e.g., survey/questionnaire
☐ Yes	☐ No	☐ N/A	Previous versions of the IRB approved study tools, e.g., survey/questionnaire Total Number:
☐ Yes	☐ No	☐ N/A	Correspondence with the IRB on file: (look for signature and date when needed for submission)
☐ Yes	☐ No	☐ N/A	Initial IRB application
☐ Yes	☐ No	☐ N/A	Continuing review(s). Total Number:
☐ Yes	☐ No	☐ N/A	Modification Request(s). Total Number:
☐ Yes	☐ No	☐ N/A	Reportable New Information form(s). Total Number:
☐ Yes	☐ No	☐ N/A	Notifications of IRB disapproval, deferral, modifications required to secure approval
☐ Yes	☐ No	☐ N/A	Responses to IRB actions
☐ Yes	☐ No	☐ N/A	IRB suspensions or terminations
☐ Yes	☐ No	☐ N/A	Copies of e-mail correspondence with the IRB
☐ Yes	☐ No	☐ N/A	Other communications with the IRB
☐ Yes	☐ No	☐ N/A	Records of investigator and study staff human research training
☐ Yes	☐ No	☐ N/A	Training certificates are valid (completed within the past 3 years or appropriate amount of time per institutional policy)
☐ Yes	☐ No	☐ N/A	CVs or other relevant documents (biosketch/resume) evidencing qualifications of PI, co-investigators, and all study personnel
☐ Yes	☐ No	☐ N/A	CVs / other relevant information have been updated within the past two years (or appropriate amount of time per institutional policy or appropriate amount of time per institutional policy)
☐ Yes	☐ No	☐ N/A	CVs / other relevant information are signed and dated
☐ Yes	☐ No	☐ N/A	Signed agreements/contracts between parties
☐ Yes	☐ No	☐ N/A	Correspondences to and from the funding agency or sponsor
☐ Yes	☐ No	☐ N/A	IRB roster
☐ Yes	☐ No	☐ N/A	Documentation of Federalwide Assurance (FWA) Number

2. Logs

☐ Yes	☐ No	☐ N/A	Participant screening log. Number screened:
☐ Yes	☐ No	☐ N/A	Participant identification code list
☐ Yes	☐ No	☐ N/A	Participant enrollment log. Number enrolled:
☐ Yes	☐ No	☐ N/A	Study Staff Signature and Delegation of Responsibility log
☐ Yes	☐ No	☐ N/A	Signature log reflects all current staff working on the study
☐ Yes	☐ No	☐ N/A	Signature log reflects all previous staff working on the study
☐ Yes	☐ No	☐ N/A	Staff working on the study are IRB approved
☐ Yes	☐ No	☐ N/A	Signature log reflects PI's signature
☐ Yes	☐ No	☐ N/A	Monitoring/auditing log. Monitoring frequency:
☐ Yes	☐ No	☐ N/A	Monitoring/auditing log includes a description of monitoring activities
☐ Yes	☐ No	☐ N/A	Record of retained body fluids / tissue samples
☐ Yes	☐ No	☐ N/A	Correspondences to and from the sponsor/CRO
☐ Yes	☐ No	☐ N/A	Letters
☐ Yes	☐ No	☐ N/A	Meeting notes
☐ Yes	☐ No	☐ N/A	Notes of telephone calls
☐ Yes	☐ No	☐ N/A	Instructions for handling of investigational product(s) and trial-related materials (if not in protocol or investigator's brochure)
☐ Yes	☐ No	☐ N/A	Decoding procedures for blinded trials
☐ Yes	☐ No	☐ N/A	Normal lab values
☐ Yes	☐ No	☐ N/A	Updates to normal lab values
☐ Yes	☐ No	☐ N/A	Lab certification (e.g. CAP, CLIA)
☐ Yes	☐ No	☐ N/A	Updates to lab certification (e.g. CAP, CLIA)
☐ Yes	☐ No	☐ N/A	Lab director's CV
☐ Yes	☐ No	☐ N/A	Updates to lab director's CV
☐ Yes	☐ No	☐ N/A	Site Initiation report/visit documentation
☐ Yes	☐ No	☐ N/A	Study close-out report/visit documentation
☐ Yes	☐ No	☐ N/A	Is there a Data Safety Monitoring Plan (DSMP) for this study?
☐ Yes	☐ No	☐ N/A	Has the DSMP been followed per the IRB approved protocol?
☐ Yes	☐ No	☐ N/A	Is there a DSMB for this study?

☐ Yes	☐ No	☐ N/A	DSMB reports, meeting minutes or indication of DSMB review/recommendations. DSMB frequency:
☐ Yes	☐ No	☐ N/A	Most recently approved sample case report forms (CRF) / Data Collection Sheets
☐ Yes	☐ No	☐ N/A	For marketed products, a package insert / product information

3. Document Retention

☐ Yes	☐ No	☐ N/A	Regulatory documentation (e.g., contents of the Regulatory Binder) are retained for at least [XXXXX] years after closing out the Human Research
☐ Yes	☐ No	☐ N/A	Records for sponsored research are retained until the sponsor authorized destruction of the records. Instructions or date of authorized destruction:

4. FDA Investigational New Drug Study-specific Records[3]

☐ Yes	☐ No	☐ N/A	Is the PI a sponsor-investigator[4] (IND holder)? Fill out section 11
☐ Yes	☐ No	☐ N/A	Is there a signed FDA Form 3674 – Certificate of Registration to ClicincalTrials.gov on file? A FDA Form 3674 should be on file for each applicable study.
☐ Yes	☐ No	☐ N/A	Is a signed Investigator Statement (Form FDA 1572) on file for each investigator involved in the study?
☐ Yes	☐ No	☐ N/A	Is documentation verifying the IND number on file (e.g. copy of IB with IND number, IND acknowledgment letter from FDA for indication under study)?

If the answer to the above question is yes, and the PI is a sponsor-investigator, please complete section 11 below.
If the answer to the above question is no, please do not complete Section 11.

☐ Yes	☐ No	☐ N/A	A signed current FDA 1572 for all clinical sites?
☐ Yes	☐ No	☐ N/A	Is there a monitor[5] for this study?
☐ Yes	☐ No	☐ N/A	Are copies of all previously conducted monitoring reports received on file?
☐ Yes	☐ No	☐ N/A	Is there a monitoring log on file for all monitoring previously conducted?
☐ Yes	☐ No	☐ N/A	Previous signed versions of FDA 1572 Total Number:
☐ Yes	☐ No	☐ N/A	A current signed financial disclosure form (Form 3454 or 3455) submitted to the sponsor from each investigator listed on the 1572 or in the Investigator Statement
☐ Yes	☐ No	☐ N/A	Has the IRB been notified for all of the research team members listed on the FDA Form 1572 or who signed an Investigator Agreement?
☐ Yes	☐ No	☐ N/A	Valid licensure for each investigator / staff member listed on the 1572

3. The Investigational New Drug (IND) application is the process through which a drug sponsor alerts the FDA of its intentions to conduct clinical studies with an investigational drug. Refer to FDA guidance about when an IND is required.

4. Sponsor-investigator is the individual who both initiates and conducts an investigation, and under whose immediate direction the investigational drug is administered or dispensed. A Sponsor-investigator is required to fulfill the responsibilities of both the Investigator and the Sponsor.

5. An individual who reviews the subject safety and protocol adherence, as stated in the protocol data and safety monitoring plan. For IND studies, this is the individual listed as the monitor in section 14 of the FDA Form 1571.

☐ Yes	☐ No	☐ N/A	Current investigator brochure or product label
☐ Yes	☐ No	☐ N/A	Previous versions of or updates to the investigator brochure
☐ Yes	☐ No	☐ N/A	There is shipping log for each drug, which captures the following:
☐ Yes	☐ No	☐ N/A	Date shipment received
☐ Yes	☐ No	☐ N/A	Shipment # from packing slip study drug
☐ Yes	☐ No	☐ N/A	Batch # / lot # / code mark
☐ Yes	☐ No	☐ N/A	Expiration date
☐ Yes	☐ No	☐ N/A	# of boxes, kits, or drugs per lot #
☐ Yes	☐ No	☐ N/A	# of bottles, vials, inhalers, or drugs per box or kit
☐ Yes	☐ No	☐ N/A	Condition of study drug shipment (Intact/damaged)
☐ Yes	☐ No	☐ N/A	Receiver's name
☐ Yes	☐ No	☐ N/A	There is an accountability log for each drug under investigation, which captures the following:
☐ Yes	☐ No	☐ N/A	Participant ID #, initials, or name
☐ Yes	☐ No	☐ N/A	Lot or kit number
☐ Yes	☐ No	☐ N/A	# Bottles, vials, etc.
☐ Yes	☐ No	☐ N/A	Amount of study drug per bottle, vial, etc.
☐ Yes	☐ No	☐ N/A	Total amount dispensed
☐ Yes	☐ No	☐ N/A	Initials
☐ Yes	☐ No	☐ N/A	Date dispensed
☐ Yes	☐ No	☐ N/A	# of bottles, vials, etc. Returned
☐ Yes	☐ No	☐ N/A	Total amount returned
☐ Yes	☐ No	☐ N/A	There is an accountability log for each drug under investigation, which captures the following:
☐ Yes	☐ No	☐ N/A	Participant ID #, initials, or name
☐ Yes	☐ No	☐ N/A	Lot or kit number
☐ Yes	☐ No	☐ N/A	# Bottles, vials, etc.
☐ Yes	☐ No	☐ N/A	Amount of study drug per bottle, vial, etc.
☐ Yes	☐ No	☐ N/A	Total amount dispensed
☐ Yes	☐ No	☐ N/A	Initials
☐ Yes	☐ No	☐ N/A	Date dispensed
☐ Yes	☐ No	☐ N/A	# of bottles, vials, etc. Returned
☐ Yes	☐ No	☐ N/A	Total amount returned
☐ Yes	☐ No	☐ N/A	Balance: number dispensed less number returned

☐ Yes	☐ No	☐ N/A	Comments: participant lost, discarded, etc.
☐ Yes	☐ No	☐ N/A	Person who dispensed the drug
☐ Yes	☐ No	☐ N/A	The investigator furnishes all reports to/from the sponsor of the drug
☐ Yes	☐ No	☐ N/A	An investigator shall promptly report to the sponsor any adverse effect that may reasonably be regarded as caused by, or probably caused by, the drug. If the adverse effect is alarming, the investigator shall report the adverse effect immediately to the sponsor and IRB

5. Study Records (IDE studies)[6]

☐ Yes	☐ No	☐ N/A	Is a signed Investigator Statement on file for each investigator involved in the study?
☐ Yes	☐ No	☐ N/A	Is documentation verifying the IDE number on file (e.g. copy of device manual with IDE number, IDE acknowledgment letter from FDA for indication under study)?
☐ Yes	☐ No	☐ N/A	Is a copy of the original IDE application to the FDA on file?
☐ Yes	☐ No	☐ N/A	Are ALL amendments to the IDE on file?
☐ Yes	☐ No	☐ N/A	Are ALL annual reports to the IDE on file?
☐ Yes	☐ No	☐ N/A	Are ALL safety reports to the IDE on file?
☐ Yes	☐ No	☐ N/A	Is ALL correspondence to the FDA on file?
☐ Yes	☐ No	☐ N/A	Is there a monitor[7] for this study?
☐ Yes	☐ No	☐ N/A	Are copies of all monitoring reports received on file?
☐ Yes	☐ No	☐ N/A	Is there a monitoring log on file?
☐ Yes	☐ No	☐ N/A	Previous versions of signed Investigator Statements Total Number:
☐ Yes	☐ No	☐ N/A	A current signed financial disclosure form submitted to the sponsor from each investigator listed in the Signed Investigator Agreement
☐ Yes	☐ No	☐ N/A	Previous versions of signed financial disclosure forms submitted to the sponsor from each investigator in the Investigator Statement
☐ Yes	☐ No	☐ N/A	Has the IRB been notified for all of the research team members listed who signed an Investigator Agreement?
☐ Yes	☐ No	☐ N/A	Valid licensure for each investigator / staff member listed on the Investigator Statement
☐ Yes	☐ No	☐ N/A	Current device manual
☐ Yes	☐ No	☐ N/A	Previous versions of or updates to the device manual Total Number:
☐ Yes	☐ No	☐ N/A	There is shipping log for each device, which captures the following
☐ Yes	☐ No	☐ N/A	Date shipment received

6. Investigational Device Exemption (IDE) allows the investigational device to be used in a clinical study in order to collect safety and effectiveness data required to support a Pre-market approval (PMA) or Pre-market Notification 510(k) submission to FDA.

7. An individual who reviews the subject safety and protocol adherence, as stated in the protocol data and safety monitoring plan. For IDE studies, this individual is identified in the investigational plan.

☐ Yes	☐ No	☐ N/A	Shipment # from packing slip study device
☐ Yes	☐ No	☐ N/A	Expiration date
☐ Yes	☐ No	☐ N/A	# of boxes, kits, or devices per lot #
☐ Yes	☐ No	☐ N/A	# of bottles or devices per box or kit
☐ Yes	☐ No	☐ N/A	Condition of study drug / device shipment (Intact/damaged)
☐ Yes	☐ No	☐ N/A	Receiver's name
☐ Yes	☐ No	☐ N/A	There is an accountability log for each device under investigation, which captures the following:
☐ Yes	☐ No	☐ N/A	Participant ID#, initials, or name
☐ Yes	☐ No	☐ N/A	Model or serial #
☐ Yes	☐ No	☐ N/A	Date used/implemented
☐ Yes	☐ No	☐ N/A	Device disposition
☐ Yes	☐ No	☐ N/A	Comments, such as malfunctions, device failure, disposition of unused devices (returned to sponsor / destroyed,) or any other pertinent information concerning the device
☐ Yes	☐ No	☐ N/A	Person who administered the device
☐ Yes	☐ No	☐ N/A	Correspondence with another investigator, an IRB, the sponsor, a monitor, or FDA, including required report
☐ Yes	☐ No	☐ N/A	Reports of unanticipated adverse device effects.
☐ Yes	☐ No	☐ N/A	Reports of withdrawal of IRB approval.
☐ Yes	☐ No	☐ N/A	Progress reports submitted to the sponsor, the monitor, and the reviewing IRB at regular intervals Total Number:
☐ Yes	☐ No	☐ N/A	Reports of deviations from the investigational plan.
☐ Yes	☐ No	☐ N/A	Reports of emergency use of the investigational device without informed consent.
☐ Yes	☐ No	☐ N/A	Final report.

6. Document Retention (IRB Policy)

☐ Yes	☐ No	☐ N/A	Regulatory documentation (e.g., contents of the Regulatory Binder) are retained for at least XXXX years after closing out the Human Research. If the Human Research is sponsored, contact the sponsor before disposing of Human Research records as there may be specific policies related to record retention. Date of Document Destruction (if known):

7. Document Retention (IND studies)

☐ Yes	☐ No	☐ N/A	An investigator retains records required to be maintained under this part for a period of 2 years following the date a marketing application is approved for the drug for the indication for which it is being investigated; or, if no application is to be filed or if the application is not approved for such indication, until 2 years after the investigation is discontinued and FDA is notified. Date of Planned Document Destruction (if known):

8. Document Retention (IDE studies)

☐ Yes	☐ No	☐ N/A	An investigator or sponsor shall maintain the records required by this subpart during the investigation and for a period of 2 years after the latter of the following two dates: The date on which the investigation is terminated or completed, or the date that the records are no longer required for purposes of supporting a premarket approval application or a notice of completion of a product development protocol. Date of Document Destruction (if known):

9. Investigator Study Conduct Responsibilities (IND studies)

☐ Yes	☐ No	☐ N/A	Investigators are responsible for the control of drugs under investigation
☐ Yes	☐ No	☐ N/A	Investigators administer the drug only to participants under their personal supervision or under the supervision of a sub-investigator responsible to the investigator
☐ Yes	☐ No	☐ N/A	Investigators do not supply the investigational drug to any person not authorized to receive it
☐ Yes	☐ No	☐ N/A	If the investigation is terminated, suspended, discontinued, or completed, investigators return the unused supplies of the drug to the sponsor, or otherwise provides for disposition of the unused supplies of the drug as authorized by the sponsor
☐ Yes	☐ No	☐ N/A	If an investigational drug is participant to the Controlled Substances Act, investigators take adequate precautions, including storage of the investigational drug in a securely locked, substantially constructed cabinet, or other securely locked, substantially constructed enclosure, access to which is limited, to prevent theft or diversion of the substance into illegal channels of distribution

10. Investigator Study Conduct Responsibilities (IDE studies)

☐ Yes	☐ No	☐ N/A	Investigators permit an investigational device to be used only with participants under the investigator's supervision
☐ Yes	☐ No	☐ N/A	Investigators do not supply an investigational device to any person not authorized to receive it
☐ Yes	☐ No	☐ N/A	Upon completion or termination of a clinical investigation or the investigator's part of an investigation, or at the sponsor's request, investigators return to the sponsor any unused device or otherwise dispose of the device as the sponsor directs
☐ Yes	☐ No	☐ N/A	If the investigation is terminated, suspended, discontinued, or completed, investigators returns the unused supplies of the drug to the sponsor, or otherwise provides for disposition of the unused supplies of the drug as authorized by the sponsor

Investigators prepare and submit the following reports to the sponsor:

☐ Yes	☐ No	☐ N/A	Any unanticipated adverse device effect occurring during an investigation. (As soon as possible, but in no event later than 10 working days after first learning of the effect unless required sooner by sponsor.)
☐ Yes	☐ No	☐ N/A	Withdrawal of approval by the reviewing IRB of the investigator's part of an investigation. (Within 5 working days unless required sooner by sponsor)
☐ Yes	☐ No	☐ N/A	Progress reports on the investigation. (At least yearly.)

☐ Yes	☐ No	☐ N/A	Any deviation from the investigational plan to protect the life or physical well-being of a participant in an emergency. (As soon as possible, but in no event later than 5 working days after the emergency occurred unless required sooner by sponsor.)
☐ Yes	☐ No	☐ N/A	Emergency use of an investigational device without obtaining informed consent (Within 5 working days after the use occurs unless required sooner by sponsor.)
☐ Yes	☐ No	☐ N/A	A final report. (Within 3 months after termination or completion of the investigation or the investigator's part of the investigation unless required sooner by sponsor.)

Investigators prepare and submit the following reports to the IRB:

☐ Yes	☐ No	☐ N/A	Any unanticipated adverse device effect occurring during an investigation. (As soon as possible, but in no event later than 5 working days after first learning of the effect.)
☐ Yes	☐ No	☐ N/A	Progress reports on the investigation. (At least yearly.)
☐ Yes	☐ No	☐ N/A	Any deviation from the investigational plan to protect the life or physical well-being of a participant in an emergency. (As soon as possible, but in no event later than 5 working days after the emergency occurred.)
☐ Yes	☐ No	☐ N/A	Emergency use of an investigational device without obtaining informed consent (Within 5 working days after the use occurs.)
☐ Yes	☐ No	☐ N/A	A final report. (Within 3 months after termination or completion of the investigation or the investigator's part of the investigation.)

11. IND Sponsor-Investigator Responsibilities/Requirements

☐ Yes	☐ No	☐ N/A	Is a copy of the Original IND application to the FDA on file?
☐ Yes	☐ No	☐ N/A	Are ALL amendments to the IND on file?
☐ Yes	☐ No	☐ N/A	Are ALL annual reports to the IND on file?
☐ Yes	☐ No	☐ N/A	Are ALL safety reports on file?
☐ Yes	☐ No	☐ N/A	Is ALL correspondence with the FDA on file?
☐ Yes	☐ No	☐ N/A	Is there a form 1571 on file to accompany all of the above FDA correspondence?
☐ Yes	☐ No	☐ N/A	Is there a Financial Disclosure Form (Form 3454 or 3455) on file for each investigator listed on the FDA Form 1572 or for each person who signed an Investigator Agreement?
☐ Yes	☐ No	☐ N/A	Is there a signed FDA Form 3674 – Certificate of Registration to ClinicalTrials.gov on file? An FDA Form 3674 should be on file for each applicable study.
☐ Yes	☐ No	☐ N/A	The investigator maintains on file information pertaining to the financial interests of clinical investigators for 2 years after the date of approval of the application
☐ Yes	☐ No	☐ N/A	The investigator selects qualified investigators
☐ Yes	☐ No	☐ N/A	The investigator provides participating investigators with the information they need to conduct an investigation properly
☐ Yes	☐ No	☐ N/A	The investigator ensures that the investigation(s) is conducted in accordance with the general investigational plan and protocols contained in the IND

☐ Yes	☐ No	☐ N/A	The investigator maintains an effective IND with respect to the investigations
☐ Yes	☐ No	☐ N/A	The investigator ensures that FDA is promptly informed of significant new adverse effects or risks with respect to the drug
☐ Yes	☐ No	☐ N/A	The investigator ensures that all participating investigators are promptly informed of significant new adverse effects or risks with respect to the drug
☐ Yes	☐ No	☐ N/A	The investigator selects only investigators qualified by training and experience as appropriate experts to investigate the drug
☐ Yes	☐ No	☐ N/A	The investigator ships investigational new drugs only to investigators participating in the investigation

Before permitting an investigator to begin participation in an investigation, the investigator obtains the following:

☐ Yes	☐ No	☐ N/A	A signed investigator statement (Form FDA-1572)
☐ Yes	☐ No	☐ N/A	A CV or other statement of qualifications (biosketch/resume) of the investigator showing the education, training, and experience that qualifies the investigator as an expert in the clinical investigation of the drug for the use under investigation
☐ Yes	☐ No	☐ N/A	Sufficient accurate financial information to allow the investigator to submit complete and accurate certification or disclosure statements
☐ Yes	☐ No	☐ N/A	The investigator selects a monitor qualified by training and experience to monitor the progress of the investigation
☐ Yes	☐ No	☐ N/A	The investigator provides each participating clinical investigator an investigator brochure
☐ Yes	☐ No	☐ N/A	The investigator ensures, as the overall investigation proceeds, that each participating investigator is informed of new observations discovered by or reported to the investigator on the drug, particularly with respect to adverse effects and safe use
☐ Yes	☐ No	☐ N/A	The investigator monitors the progress of all clinical investigations being conducted under the IND
☐ Yes	☐ No	☐ N/A	If the investigator discovers that an investigator is not complying with the signed agreement (Form FDA-1572), the general investigational plan, or other applicable requirements; the investigator promptly either secures compliance or discontinues shipment of the investigational new drug to the investigator and ends the investigator's participation in the investigation
☐ Yes	☐ No	☐ N/A	If the investigator's participation in the investigation is ended, the investigator ensures that the investigator dispose of or returns the investigational drug and notifies the FDA
☐ Yes	☐ No	☐ N/A	The investigator reviews and evaluates the evidence relating to the safety and effectiveness of the drug as it is obtained from the investigator(s)

If the investigator determines that the investigational drug presents an unreasonable and significant risk to participants, the investigator:

☐ Yes	☐ No	☐ N/A	Ensures discontinuation of those investigations that present the risk
☐ Yes	☐ No	☐ N/A	Notifies the FDA, all institutional review boards, and all investigators who have at any time participated in the investigation of the discontinuance
☐ Yes	☐ No	☐ N/A	Ensures the disposition of all stocks of the drug outstanding

☐ Yes	☐ No	☐ N/A	Furnishes the FDA with a full report of the investigator's actions
☐ Yes	☐ No	☐ N/A	The investigator maintains adequate records showing the receipt, shipment, or other disposition of the investigational drug, including, as appropriate, the name of the investigator to whom the drug is shipped, and the date, quantity, and batch or code mark of each such shipment
☐ Yes	☐ No	☐ N/A	The investigator retains these records and reports for 2 years after a marketing application is approved for the drug; or, if an application is not approved for the drug, until 2 years after shipment and delivery of the drug for investigational use is discontinued and FDA has been so notified
☐ Yes	☐ No	☐ N/A	The investigator retains reserve samples of any test article and reference standard identified in, and used in any bioequivalence or bioavailability studies and release the reserve samples to the FDA upon request
☐ Yes	☐ No	☐ N/A	The investigator retains each reserve sample for a period of at least 5 years following the date on which the application or supplemental application is approved, or, if such application or supplemental application is not approved, at least 5 years following the date of completion of the bioavailability study
☐ Yes	☐ No	☐ N/A	The investigator permits, upon request from any properly authorized officer or employee of the Food and Drug Administration, at reasonable times, such officer or employee to have access to and copy and verify any records and reports relating to a clinical investigation being conducted under the IND
☐ Yes	☐ No	☐ N/A	The investigator submits, upon written request by the FDA, the records or reports (or copies of them) to the FDA
☐ Yes	☐ No	☐ N/A	The investigator discontinues shipments of the drug to any investigator who has failed to maintain or make available records or reports of the investigation as required

If an investigational new drug is a substance listed in any schedule of the Controlled Substances Act (21 U.S.C. 801; 21 CFR part 1308), the investigator ensures:

☐ Yes	☐ No	☐ N/A	Upon the request of a properly authorized employee of the Drug Enforcement Administration of the U.S. Department of Justice, all records concerning shipment, delivery, receipt, and disposition of the drug, which are required to be kept be made available by the investigator to whom the request is made, for inspection and copying
☐ Yes	☐ No	☐ N/A	That adequate precautions are taken, including storage of the investigational drug in a securely locked, substantially constructed cabinet, or other securely locked, substantially constructed enclosure, access to which is limited, to prevent theft or diversion of the substance into illegal channels of distribution
☐ Yes	☐ No	☐ N/A	The investigator ensures the return of all unused supplies of the investigational drug from each individual investigator whose participation in the investigation is discontinued or terminated

PARTICIPANT FILES

(Complete for sample of enrolled participants. If participant files are not accessible, disregard this section.)

Principal Investigator	
Protocol # / Study Title	
Total Sample Reviewed	
Participant IDs	
Name of Person Completing Checklist	
Date Completed	

1. Recruitment

☐ Yes	☐ No	☐ N/A	Are all the recruitment methods/processes being followed in accordance with the IRB approved protocol?
☐ Yes	☐ No	☐ N/A	Have ALL recruitment materials (e.g., advertisements and telephone scripts) been approved by the IRB? Note: All recruitment materials must be approved prior to use and must be reapproved at the time of continuing review.

2. Participant Selection

☐ Yes	☐ No	☐ N/A	Is source documentation on file to verify inclusion/exclusion criteria?
☐ Yes	☐ No	☐ N/A	There is a completed eligibility checklist
☐ Yes	☐ No	☐ N/A	The eligibility criteria checklist includes dated signature/initials of the person making the eligibility determination
☐ Yes	☐ No	☐ N/A	For participants who did not meet eligibility (e.g. screen-failures), identifiable information was destroyed or authorization was obtained to keep participant information

3. Consent

☐ Yes	☐ No	☐ N/A	Was the consent process conducted per the IRB-approved protocol?
☐ Yes	☐ No	☐ N/A	The number of participants who have signed consent forms, i.e., enrolled, is no greater than the IRB-approved sample size / enrollment
☐ Yes	☐ No	☐ N/A	Investigators obtained consent from each participant prior to the start of any study procedures
☐ Yes	☐ No	☐ N/A	Original copies (not photo copies) of all consent forms signed and dated by participants are on file
☐ Yes	☐ No	☐ N/A	Valid IRB-approved consent forms were used
☐ Yes	☐ No	☐ N/A	All pages of the consent forms are on file for each participant
☐ Yes	☐ No	☐ N/A	All yes/no, checkboxes, or similar options on the consent forms are completed and/or initialed

☐ Yes	☐ No	☐ N/A	Consent forms are free of any handwritten changes or corrections
☐ Yes	☐ No	☐ N/A	The participant / participant representative signed his/her own consent forms (Exceptions: IRB-approved surrogate)
☐ Yes	☐ No	☐ N/A	The participant / participant representative received a copy of the consent form
☐ Yes	☐ No	☐ N/A	The participant's / participant representative's receipt of a copy of the consent form is documented, e.g., Enrollment Log
☐ Yes	☐ No	☐ N/A	An IRB-approved study representative obtained consent for all participants
☐ Yes	☐ No	☐ N/A	An IRB-approved study representative signed/dated the consent form
☐ Yes	☐ No	☐ N/A	An IRB-approved study representative entered the same date as the participant / participant representative on the consent form
☐ Yes	☐ No	☐ N/A	Were non-English speaking subjects enrolled?
☐ Yes	☐ No	☐ N/A	If non-English speaking subjects were enrolled, was the IRB-approved process for enrolling non-English speaking subjects followed?
☐ Yes	☐ No	☐ N/A	If Short Form Consent is implemented, a witness signed and dated the consent form
☐ Yes	☐ No	☐ N/A	Consent is obtained from enrolled minors that reach local age of majority during the study
☐ Yes	☐ No	☐ N/A	Waiver of the requirement to obtain consent and/or alteration of consent process on file
☐ Yes	☐ No	☐ N/A	Wavier of documentation (signature requirement) on file

4. Prompt Reporting Requirements

☐ Yes	☐ No	☐ N/A	All prompt reporting requirements have been fulfilled

5. Data Collection Source Documents

☐ Yes	☐ No	☐ N/A	Data collection complete/accurate for each participant. (e.g., no blank fields / missing data)
☐ Yes	☐ No	☐ N/A	Source documentation is available to support data entry
☐ Yes	☐ No	☐ N/A	The source documentation / CRF for each participant includes dated signature/initials of the person obtaining the information for each participant (i.e. physical or clinical assessment pages)
☐ Yes	☐ No	☐ N/A	Changes/cross-outs, additional comments (if any) in participant files routinely initialed and dated
☐ Yes	☐ No	☐ N/A	For any changes/cross-outs being made, the original entry is still legible. (e.g., use of white-out or pencil erased entries is not acceptable)

6. Drug/Device Dispensing Accountability (for non-investigational drugs, biologics, devices)

Note: This section may not apply to your study if an investigational product, or "test article," is not part of the study. If that is the case, Check "N/A" in section 6.

Who is responsible for drug/device accountability?
☐ Study Site   ☐ Research Pharmacy   ☐ Other: ☐ N/A

If study site is responsible for drug/device accountability, complete the section below.

☐ Yes	☐ No	☐ N/A	Is documentation on file for receipt of the investigational product?
☐ Yes	☐ No	☐ N/A	Is there documentation of drug/biologic/device use for each subject (e.g., drug accountability log, study file notation)?
☐ Yes	☐ No	☐ N/A	Is there documentation of return of drug/biologic/device from the subject to the study site?
☐ Yes	☐ No	☐ N/A	Is there documentation of the return of the drug to the sponsor / manufacturer / research pharmacy or documentation of the destruction of the drug / biologic device?
☐ Yes	☐ No	☐ N/A	Have there been any other events (e.g., drug/biologic dosing errors or device malfunctions) to date?
☐ Yes	☐ No	☐ N/A	Have the events been reported to the IRB as unanticipated problems?

7. Laboratory Documentation

Note: This section may not apply to your study if an investigational product, or "test article," is not part of the study. If that is the case, Check "N/A" in section 7.

☐ Yes	☐ No	☐ N/A	Is Laboratory Certification (CLIA/CAP) current and on file?
☐ Yes	☐ No	☐ N/A	Are all out-of-range laboratory values marked as to their clinical significance?
☐ Yes	☐ No	☐ N/A	Are laboratory reference ranges (normal values) on file?

External Audit Prep Checklist

Instructions: Use the first two pages of this checklist to record information provided by the auditor at the time of initial contact. The remainder of the document should be used to track the progress of the pre-inspection preparation tasks. Check each item as it is completed and record pertinent comments.

Initial Audit Notification

Notification Date:	Visit Start Date:
Estimated Time of Arrival:	Expected Duration:

Auditor's Contact Information:	Name:
	Telephone:
	Title:
Additional Auditors' Names:	

Protocol Information

Protocol Number(s):	Details:
Principal Investigator:	
Co-Investigator(s):	

Reason for inspection

☐ Routine (not-for-cause)	Details:
☐ Directed (for-cause)	
☐ Follow-up (e.g., 483; warning letters)	
☐ Other:	Details:

Personnel Requested by Inspector (Use a separate sheet if needed)

Who:	When:

Documents Requested by Inspector (Use a separate sheet if needed)

Document requested (Check box if document requested prior to inspection)	Document requested (Check box if document requested prior to inspection)
☐	☐
☐	☐
☐	☐
☐	☐
☐	☐
☐	☐
☐	☐
☐	☐
☐	☐
☐	☐
☐	☐
☐	☐

Shipping/Delivery information for documents requested prior to the inspection visit

Name of Recipient:	Delivery Date:
Address:	☐ Overnight
	☐ Registered
	☐ Certified
E-mail:	☐ Courier

Delivery Details:

Please document any other details from the initial contact not noted above:

Administrative

	Task	Yes (Done/ Available)	No (Provide comment)	Comments
Notify all parties of impending inspection	Sponsor	☐	☐	
	IRB/EC	☐	☐	
	Quality Improvement Program	☐	☐	
	Principal Investigator	☐	☐	
	Sub-Investigator(s)	☐	☐	
	Study Coordinator(s)	☐	☐	
	Pharmacy (if applicable)	☐	☐	
	Laboratory(ies)	☐	☐	
	Medical Records	☐	☐	
	Legal Counsel	☐	☐	
	Other (specify in comments)	☐	☐	
Review Internal SOPs	IRB Policies, Department SOPs, Research Protocol	☐	☐	
Identify work space for the Inspector	Conference room/office	☐	☐	
	Telephone	☐	☐	
	Copier	☐	☐	
Review staff schedules	Review staff schedules to ensure staff availability (vacations, appointments, miscellaneous time off, etc.)	☐	☐	
	Reschedule non-essential visits/ meetings if possible	☐	☐	

Regulatory Documents

	Task	Yes (Done/ Available)	No (Provide comment)	Comments
Locate, compile, organize, and review documents for accuracy and completeness	Note: Use QIP's Investigator Self-Assessment checklist as a guide for conducting internal review of study regulatory files	☐	☐	

Administrative

Notes:

Labs and External Clinical Sites

	Task	Yes (Done/ Available)	No (Provide comment)	Comments
Locate, compile, organize, and review documents for accuracy and completeness	Investigational agent accountability logs and are on file, complete and accurate	☐	☐	
	Specimen logs are on file, complete and accurate	☐	☐	
	Ordering/shipping receipts on file	☐	☐	
	Copies of laboratory audits, action plans, and corrective action reports	☐	☐	
	Temperature logs for applicable equipment (refrigerators, freezers, storage cabinets, etc.)	☐	☐	
	Calibration and maintenance records for all laboratory equipment (if applicable)	☐	☐	
	Other (please add any additional site-specific pharmacy documents below)	☐	☐	

Notes:

Delegation of Responsibility Log

Instructions: Use this log to document all study personnel and their specific responsibilities, signatures, and dates of obligation during the study.

Investigator Name: _____ Study Title / Number: _____ Site Number: _____

Print Name	Signature	Initials	Dates of Responsibility*		Delegated Responsibilities**	PI Initial/Date
			Start	End		

*Start date should be the date of IRB approval of study personnel.

**Enter number(s) that corresponds to the responsibilities: (1) obtain informed consent (2) source document completion (3) case report form (CRF) completion (4) assess inclusion and exclusion criteria (5) physical examination (6) obtain medical history (7) obtain medication history (8) administer investigational drug (IP) (9) dispense IP (10) laboratory specimen collection/shipment (12) adverse event inquiry and reporting (13) Other _____

I certify that the above individuals are appropriately trained, have read the protocol and pertinent sections of 21CFR 50 and 56 and ICH GCPs, and are authorized to perform the above study-related tasks/procedures. Although I have delegated significant trial-related duties, as the principal investigator, I still maintain full responsibility for this trial.

Investigator Signature: _____ Date: _____

Human Research Training Log

Investigator Name:	Study Title/Number:	Site Number:

Name	Signature	Title of Training	Date of Training

Investigational Device Accountability Log

Investigator Name:

Device Name:

Study Title/Number:

Site Number

Date Received	Model #	Serial #	Lot No.	Participant ID	Date(s) Used	Indicate: Returned, Destroyed, Repaired	Date Returned, Destroyed, Repaired	Study Staff Initials	Comments

Investigational Drug Accountability Log: Subject Record

Investigator Name:

Name of Drug:

Study Title/Number:

Site Number

Date	Subject ID Number	Subject's Initials	Dose	Quantity Dispensed and/or Received	Balance Forward / Balance	Lot No.	Recorder's Initials
21 Mar 2018	115	XYZ	100mg	50 tabs	200 / 150	39999	ABC

Reportable New Information Log

Investigator Name: _____

Study Title/Number: _____

Site Number: _____

Date event became known to study staff	Description of Event	RNI Category* (see chart)	Risk or Harm Classification** (see chart)	Date IRB Notified (if applicable)	Date Sponsor Notified (if applicable)	PI Initial and Date

*RNI Category — use appropriate RNI category letter code in log (include all that apply)

**RNI Classification — use appropriate risk or harm classification number code in log (include all that apply)

* RNI CATEGORY

A. Noncompliance: Noncompliance with the federal regulations governing human research or with the requirements or determinations of the IRB, or an allegation of such noncompliance.

B. Audit: Audit, inspection, or inquiry by a federal agency.

C. Report: Written reports of study monitors.

D. Researcher Error: Failure to follow the protocol due to the action or inaction of the investigator or research staff.

E. Confidentiality: Breach of confidentiality.

F. Unreviewed Change: Change to the protocol taken without prior IRB review to eliminate an apparent immediate hazard to a subject.

G. Incarceration: Incarceration of a subject in a study not approved by the IRB to involve prisoners.

H. Complaint: Complaint of a subject that cannot be resolved by the research team.

I. Suspension: Premature suspension or termination of the research by the sponsor, investigator, or institution.

J. Unanticipated Adverse Device Effect: Any serious adverse effect on health or safety or any life-threatening problem or death caused by, or associated with, a device, if that effect, problem, or death was not previously identified in nature, severity, or degree of incidence in the investigational plan or application (including a supplementary plan or application), or any other unanticipated serious problem associated with a device that relates to the rights, safety, or welfare of subjects.

K. VA-SAE: For Department of Veterans Affairs (VA) research, all local or internal serious adverse events (SAEs).

** RISK OR HARM CATEGORY

1. **Risk:** Information that indicates a new or increased risk or safety issue such as:

   1.1. New Information (e.g., an interim analysis, safety monitoring report, publication in the literature, sponsor report, or investigator finding) that indicates an increase in the frequency or magnitude of a previously known risk or uncovers a new risk.

   1.2. Investigator brochure, package insert, or device labeling is revised to indicate an increase in the frequency or magnitude of a previously known risk, or to describe a new risk.

   1.3. Withdrawal, restriction, or modification of a marketed approval of a drug, device, or biologic used in a research protocol.

   1.4. Protocol violation that harmed subjects or others or that indicates subjects or others might be at increased risk of harm.

   1.5. Complaint of a subject that indicates subjects or others might be at increased risk of harm or at risk of a new harm.

   1.6. Any changes significantly affecting the conduct of the research.

2. **Harm:** Any harm experienced by a subject or other individual that, in the opinion of the investigator, is unexpected and at least possibly related to the research procedures.

   2.1. A harm is *"unexpected"* when its specificity or severity is inconsistent with risk information previously reviewed and approved by the IRB in terms of nature, severity, frequency, and characteristics of the study population.

   2.2. A harm is *"possibly related"* to the research procedures if, in the opinion of the investigator, the research procedures more likely than not caused the harm.

Site Screening and Enrollment Log

Instructions: Use this log to list participants screened and include those who failed screening and those who are enrolled.

Investigator Name:			Study Title/Number:		Site Number	
Participant ID	Date of Consent	Version of Consent	Date Screened	Eligible for Enrollment? (Y/N)	Ineligibility Reason (if applicable)	

Study Monitoring / Site Visit Log

Investigator Name:	Study Title/Number:	Site Number
Name	Signature	Purpose of Visit	Date of Visit

Bibliography

Preface

Institute of Medicine. *Crossing the Quality Chasm: A New Health System for the 21st Century*. Washington, DC: National Academies Press, 2001, 232.

Chapter 1: Introduction to Quality Assurance and Quality Improvement Programs

Association for the Accreditation of Human Research Protection Programs, Inc. (AAHRPP). http://www.aahrpp.org.

———. "AAHRPP Evaluation Instrument." Last modified July 13, 2018. https://admin .aahrpp.org/_layouts/15/download.aspx?SourceUrl=/Website%20Documents /AAHRPP%20Evaluation%20Instrument%20(2018-07-13)%20published.pdf.

Office for Human Research Protections. "International Program." https://www.hhs.gov /ohrp/international/index.html.

———. "Objectives and Overview of the OHRP Quality Improvement Program." Accessed July 8, 2015. http://archive.hhs.gov/ohrp/humansubjects/qip/qipdesc.pdf (site discontinued).

———. "OHRP QA Self-Assessment Tool." Last modified March 18, 2016. https://www .hhs.gov/ohrp/education-and-outreach/human-research-protection-program -fundamentals/ohrp-self-assessment-tool/index.html.

University of Pittsburgh, Education & Compliance Office for Human Subject Research. Last modified November 6, 2016. http://www.ecohsr.pitt.edu/about.

U.S. Department of Health and Human Services. "Policy for Protection of Human Research Subjects." Last modified January 15, 2010. https://www.hhs.gov/ohrp /regulations-and-policy/regulations/common-rule/index.html.

———. "Summary of the HIPAA Privacy Rule." https://www.hhs.gov/hipaa/for-profes sionals/privacy/laws-regulations/index.html.

U.S. Food and Drug Administration. "Regulations: Good Clinical Practice and Clinical Trials." Last modified March 30, 2018. https://www.fda.gov/ScienceResearch /SpecialTopics/RunningClinicalTrials/ucm155713.htm.

Chapter 2: Types of QA/QI Programs

Emanuel, E. *The Concept of Conflicts of Interest*. New York: Oxford Textbook of Clinical Research Ethics, 2008, 758–766.

Chapter 3: Policies and Procedures

Alion Science and Technology. "Alion HRPP Accreditation Standards." Accessed May 26, 2018. http://www.alionhrpp.com/accreditation-services-/standards.

Association for the Accreditation of Human Research Protection Programs, Inc. "AAHRPP

Domain I: Organization." Accessed May 26, 2018. http://www.aahrpp.org/apply
/web-document-library/domain-i-organization.

Chapter 4: Investigator Site Review

U.S. Food and Drug Administration. "E6(R2) Good Clinical Practice: Integrated Addendum to ICH E6(R1) Guidance for Industry." Updated March 2018. https://www.fda
.gov/regulatory-information/search-fda-guidance-documents/e6r2-good-clinical
-practice-integrated-addendum-ich-e6r1.

Chapter 5: Evaluating IRB Compliance

Office for Human Research Protections. "45 CFR 46 Protection of Human Subjects." Last
modified January 15, 2010. https://www.hhs.gov/ohrp/regulations-and-policy
/regulations/45-cfr-46/index.html.
———— "Institutional Review Board Written Procedures: Guidance for Institutions and
IRBs." Last modified May 2018. https://www.hhs.gov/ohrp/regulations-and-policy
/guidance/institutional-issues/institutional-review-board-written-procedures/index
.html.
———— "Minutes of Institutional Review Board Meetings Guidance for Institutions and
IRBs." Last modified September 2017. https://www.hhs.gov/ohrp/minutes-institu
tional-review-board-irb-meetings-guidance-institutions-and-irbs.html-0.
U.S. Food and Drug Administration. "21 CFR 56 FDA Regulations Institutional Review
Boards." Last modified April 1, 2017. http://www.accessdata.fda.gov/scripts/cdrh
/cfdocs/cfcfr/CFRSearch.cfm?CFRPart=56.

Chapter 6: Metrics and Communicating Observations of Noncompliance

Association for the Accreditation of Human Research Protection Programs, Inc.
"AAHRPP Annual Report." Last modified May 9, 2018. http://www.aahrpp.org
/apply/maintaining-accreditation/annual-reports.

Index